# Understanding TEENAGE ANXIETY

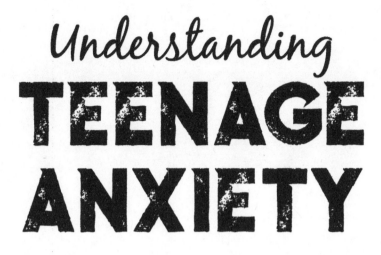

# Understanding TEENAGE ANXIETY

## A Parent's Guide to Improving Your Teen's Mental Health

Jennifer Browne & Cody Buchanan

Skyhorse Publishing

Skyhorse Publishing books may be purchased in bulk at special discounts for sales promotion, corporate gifts, fund-raising, or educational purposes. Special editions can also be created to specifications. For details, contact the Special Sales Department, Skyhorse Publishing, 307 West 36th Street, 11th Floor, New York, NY 10018 or info@skyhorsepublishing.com.



Visit our website at www.skyhorsepublishing.com.

10 9 8 7 6 5 4 3 2 1

Library of Congress Cataloging-in-Publication Data is available on file.

Cover design by Peter Donahue
Cover illustration by iStockphoto

Print ISBN: 978-1-5107-4365-6
Ebook ISBN: 978-1-5107-4366-3

Printed in the United States of America

This book is for everyone who is currently as confused and scared as we were—both caregivers and teenagers alike.

Learning to understand teenage anxiety—anxiety in general—is a journey. It takes a ton of patience and hard work, but resources are available. And although you may not feel like it right now, inhale deeply, exhale slowly, and know that you're not alone, you're loved, and everything will be okay.

# CONTENTS

"Anxiety disorders affect 25.1% of children between thirteen and eighteen years old. Research shows that untreated children with anxiety disorders are at higher risk to perform poorly in school, miss out on important social experiences, and engage in substance abuse."[1]

# FOREWORD

PARENTS today are raising children during what can only be described as a veritable epidemic of anxiety. One in five of us will be clinically diagnosable at some point in our lifetime. And approximately 75 percent of kids struggling with anxiety will never receive direct support from a qualified provider. This means that as parents, you will be the primary source of healing for your child.

That might sound pretty daunting, but as you are about to discover in this book, it is doable—and *exactly* as nature intended it to be. It turns out that this anxiety epidemic might actually be serving as a giant wake-up call for parents everywhere to know the true power in raising your kids to live life as was uniquely intended for them.

One of the amazing aspects of Jennifer and Cody's collaborative effort is in shining a light on the parents' key role. It has long been my belief that parents are the *true* experts on their children. Period. I have seen this play out hundreds of times in my clinical practice and live it every day in my life as a mom to two adolescents of my own.

Watching your child struggle and shut down can be a terrifying experience, and it might be very difficult to hang on to your parent "swagger" along the way. But it is exactly that swagger, the ability to step in and provide from a combined place of intuition and knowledge, that is going to get your child through this. There *is* a way through, and you really are the vehicle through which that path will be illuminated.

Especially important when supporting your anxious teen and covered in a way that is at once complex, direct, and distilled in this book is a foundational respect for child development. When we as parents can make sense of how the brain develops and what allows brains to thrive, we are well positioned to set up our children's world and respond to their needs in supportive ways.

It turns out that the human brain is not fully developed until sometime in the mid- to late twenties. (A little earlier for females, and a little later for males.) Knowing that teenagers are not young adults or even capable of approximating adult-like self-regulation and all that goes with that allows us to see them as who they really are: children. Yes, they walk around in adult-like bodies with a lot of adult-like capabilities like driving and getting a job. But this adult-like facade betrays the fact that their brains still have *years* of maturing to do before they will be scientifically and otherwise defined as "fully developed." The bottom line? Don't retire too soon from your role as a deeply involved, fully present, and completely attuned parent to your teen—a message that is echoed brilliantly throughout the pages of this book.

And finally, my favorite part of this book came from the weaving together of two life paths and the illustration of both Cody's and Jennifer's individual growth on their overlapping journeys. It is my very firm belief that we are all on this planet to become the best versions of ourselves in this lifetime. That can look really different from one person to the next and involves very unique lessons and learning.

If you are a parent of a child struggling with anxiety, make no mistake that you are being handed a gift, a powerful opportunity to step fully into who you are. As hard as it can be to fathom this, know that anxiety can be a gift to your child, too. With your support and a tenacious amount of swagger, your child is also being given a powerful opportunity to step fully into who he or she is . . . *because of anxiety.*

You will hear through the language and writing of both Jennifer and Cody that anxiety leads to incredible personal growth and an actualizing of remarkable potential. I daresay Jennifer and Cody have truly stepped in. The sky is the limit. And so too can it be that way for you.

You've got this. Now, read on.

Dr. Vanessa Lapointe, R. Psych.
—author of *Discipline without Damage*
and *Parenting Right from the Start*

# INTRODUCTION

IT'S two o'clock in the afternoon on a Friday, and I'm trying to wake my eighteen-year-old son for the fifth time today. He's ignored every attempt so far, so I decide to take it up a notch and snatch his phone—his lifeline—from the windowsill by his bed—a bed that hasn't been made by him in over a year.

This gets his attention.

I calmly state that unless he's fully clothed and upstairs in two minutes, he's losing the phone for the weekend, and predictably, this enrages him. He makes his way upstairs in the allotted amount of time, but he's emotionally charged, and I know from previous experience that this won't go well for either of us. Forty-five minutes later, I've collected my laptop (which he'd taken and threatened to shatter on the sidewalk), and he's in the shower because it might be the only opportunity he gets to clean himself for the next few days—he doesn't like to shower at friends' houses.

I've asked him to leave the house indefinitely for the third time in six months . . . but let's back up.

Three years prior to writing this book, this lonely, confused, angry teenager was a fifteen-year-old kid who routinely raked in great grades, had good friends, participated in organized sports, and attended family functions. He was looking forward to attaining his driver's license and spoke enthusiastically about scoring himself his first job. For all intents and purposes, he was a happy, healthy, intelligent kid whose kind and polite demeanor was regularly complimented by other parents. Sure, he had minor obsessive-compulsive tendencies (who doesn't?), but that was the only hint of the mental health decline to come—and it came hard and fast.

Within a year, his grades fell rapidly, so much so that by his final year of high school, he didn't stand a chance—he didn't graduate. Not because he wasn't bright enough to pass his exams, but because he couldn't physically make his way into the classroom without subjecting himself to an onslaught of panic attacks.

He began to self-medicate by abusing drugs that let him avoid uncomfortable situations and prescription medication that his friends gave him. Almost his entire social network was medicated by their family physicians, so narcotics like Adderall, Xanax, Ativan, and Valium were made available to him whenever he wanted them. Creating various cocktails consisting of these medications became a way to pass the time.

He became too paralyzed to drive. A simple lesson would entice migraines, nausea, and immediate exhaustion.

At this point, I was embarrassed because I'd witnessed most of my friends' teens graduate, move away to attend various universities, or at the very least manage to hold down a full-time job. I didn't understand why my kid was different and tried very hard not to label him as being simply lazy, but it was extremely difficult not to do that: it's exactly what it looked like. Scenes from the movie *Failure to Launch* danced around my head, and I decided tough love needed to be implemented in the game plan, but this approach only made it worse.

He slept in every day. He craved sugar and simple carbohydrates on a whole other level. He consumed energy drinks as one would water. Unlike other people his age, he wasn't interested in drinking alcohol, because booze is a depressant—he wanted stimulants because he was desperate to do something—anything—that would help him fill the day with activity and make him feel like he'd been productive.

There was a lot of anger.

He witnessed his friends doing things they love, paying for cool experiences with the cash they'd made at their jobs—jobs that he didn't think he could get. He didn't even apply; the thought of taking an interview was enough to make his heart beat, hands get clammy, and head pound. I tried to tell him these are normal symptoms for somebody to experience when they're nervous, and that it was okay, but then he'd fall into hours of research that led him to believe he was having a heart attack or a brain aneurysm or worse.

Maybe brain cancer.

As a single parent, and especially because I gave birth to him at the same age he is now, I blamed myself for taking on a responsibility that I clearly couldn't handle—I screwed up. I messed up one of the humans I love most.

He routinely had fits of rage that resulted in a plethora of hurtful accusations and cursing, holes in drywall, bloodied knuckles, tears. I tried to reason and forgive, but eventually, I deemed these fits unsafe to be around, for both myself and my other children—I became scared of my own kid and *for* my own kid.

I imagined him living on the street (he already looked like he did; he hadn't shaved or cut his hair in months, and he rotated through the same two or three T-shirts), and the thought of him self-medicating with something lethal but cheap and readily available like fentanyl was enough to disrupt my sleep for months. We'd attended a funeral around this time for good friends who lost their son to a fentanyl overdose, and I was completely terrified.

He's six feet one and weighed, at the height of his anxiety, approximately 120 pounds. (For reference, the bottom range of a normal body mass index [BMI] for his height is 143 pounds; a healthy BMI would be closer to between 165 and 185.)

He talked about suicide. While accompanying him to a doctor's appointment where he was trying hard to sell the physician on prescribing him his choice of stimulants, the doctor asked if he would kill himself if there were a magic button he could push that would end his life immediately and painlessly.

With zero hesitation, he said yes.

By this time, he and I clearly had a codependent, unhealthy, rapidly worsening cycle of communication, and neither of us knew how to break it. He wouldn't see a therapist, wouldn't take the selective serotonin reuptake inhibitors (SSRIs) that were prescribed to him for anxiety and depression because he couldn't get through the first few weeks of side effects, and wouldn't put himself on a healthy sleep schedule. I tried exploring various coping mechanisms that might have been of help to him, suggesting dietary changes, aromatherapy, yoga, and meditation.

He refused to want to try anything but what I (and the various doctors he'd seen) perceived to be bandage solutions—medications that gave him instant relief from his symptoms but did nothing for long-term behavior management. I couldn't force him to do anything he didn't want to do—and that included ceasing methods of self-harm such as head banging. I didn't know if he was cutting; some of his friends did that.

And guess what? Millions of parents are in the same situation I was in *right now.*

Is it a millennial mindset? Is it the culture of anxiety we've been fostering and cultivating for the past decade? Is it inept parenting? Or was—is—my kid legitimately mentally unwell?

Does he *actually* suffer from depression, anxiety, and/or attention deficit hyperactivity disorder (ADHD)? And if he does, how do I help him when I'm trying to reason with a teenage brain that does not compute because "you don't know what this is like?"

If you can relate to this experience in any way, this book was written for you.

## Let's Get Personal

I am not a doctor or psychologist; I have no formal education on the topic of anxiety. What I *do* have are years of experience that have literally changed my life and inspired me to want to share what I've learned with others.

Learning how to navigate my son (and the rest of our family) through his chronic, debilitating anxiety was one of the hardest things I've ever had to do in my whole life. My husband of thirteen years and I divorced during these years, and the stress that resulted from that experience didn't come close to the stress I sustained while trying to keep Cody mentally stable enough to not hurt himself or others. I've never been so scared. *Ever.*

I've also never felt so empowered as I do now, postcrisis, with a plethora of knowledge under my belt that was collected piece by piece during some of the darkest days of my life.

The most useful lesson I've learned from my experience in trying (and, in the earlier years, mostly failing) to help my anxious son is this: you can't *fix* anxiety itself, but the way you respond to it can help a great deal. Your child begins to heal and cope when you learn to respond in very specific ways to his plight. And there's a huge relief in what I'm about to reveal next:

you don't have to *actually* understand anxiety; you only have to acknowledge it, be patient with it, and learn out how to respond to it in a way that is both helpful and nurturing. That is what this book intends to do—empower you to understand why responding to your teen's anxiety in a certain way is important and then give you tools to help your son or daughter feel better, learn to cope, and start living fulfilling lives again.

There are two basic components to this book. The first component is all about understanding what teenage anxiety is, understanding what your teen may be dealing with in regard to living with chronic anxiety, and learning to craft appropriate, supportive, and nurturing responses to their various predicaments.

The second component involves educating yourself on various coping mechanisms to share and further craft or personalize with your teen so that they may better take control of their anxiety and participate fully in their own life.

We're going to discuss the question of why in relation to anxiety, and cover topics such as adolescent brain development, common anxiety disorders, and relationships with caregivers. We'll also talk about how we can improve symptoms and begin to pave a healthier path, with topics that cover supportive coping mechanisms, the importance of improving gut health, and ways for you—the caregiver—to examine your own self-care throughout the process.

But that's not all.

Cody weighs in periodically on his experiences from a teenager's perspective and shares what he's learned and what he found most difficult in his own journey to control his anxious life. While it's always helpful to talk to other parents or doctors about your teen's anxiety, it's also refreshing and necessary to jump into the mind of a teen who's gone through it.

Each of the twelve chapters will conclude with solid ideas on what we can actively do as family members to improve the issues that were highlighted in the previous pages. Once we're open to why our teens may be suffering with anxiety and how to help them feel energized and hopeful again, things will start to change, peace will be restored, and everyone will get their lives back.

I promise.

*We* promise.

# 1

# AN ANXIOUS GENERATION

> "Up to 25% of thirteen to eighteen-year-olds will have an anxiety disorder at some point."
>
> —National Institute of Mental Health

WE live in anxious times.

There is more competition for education than ever before. When my father became a policeman in 1987, he only needed a character referral. Nowadays, a degree in criminology might get your foot in the door of a local detachment, but not always. And a full-time teaching position? One is required to hold an undergraduate degree with a teachable major, as well as a professional development certification to secure this type of employment. That's at least five years of undergraduate school in order to start earning approximately forty thousand dollars a year to start.

What about obtaining those degrees to begin with? Competition is fierce. Simply scoring great grades and volunteering somewhere strategic for a couple of months doesn't guarantee you anything anymore. My kids' babysitter had a bigger, better, more impressive portfolio than I currently do by the time she was eighteen.

Life for teens is *competitive.*

Dr. Suniya Luthar, a psychology professor at Arizona State University, observes, "There's always one more activity, one more A.P. class, one more thing to do to get into a top college. Kids have a sense that they're not measuring up. The pressure is relentless and getting worse."[1]

In fact, experts say teens are growing up with more anxiety and less self-esteem than ever before.

"Teens and their parents are recognizing that anxiety disorders can be serious, and they are beginning to advocate for treatment at a level that far surpasses care-seeking a generation ago. Anxiety is the number one cause for concern at college counseling services."[2]

## What Is Anxiety?

*Anxiety* is a word or term that's become much more popular in the last decade or so. When I was in high school, no one ever talked about anxiety, let alone knew several peers who were suffering from the same affliction. Now I hear it all the time, and it's become a mainstream term among teens, especially.

But what exactly is it?

In short (because we really dig into this throughout the entire book), *anxiety* is a term used to describe a specific set of symptoms that negatively affect the way the sufferer is able to live their life. The word is often synonymous with stress and depression, and it operates on a huge scale. For example, preparing for a job interview can give people mild feelings of anxiety, but the word is also used to describe the mental state that one is engulfed in when they literally cannot function due to ongoing and unfounded fears. And for those who live with the disorder at this kind of level, chronic anxiety becomes something to fear itself.

In Dr. Peter Breggin's book *Guilt, Shame, and Anxiety*, he writes, "Anxiety encourages us to be helpless."[3] It gives messages such as these:

- That's too challenging to face.
- Don't try and think about that; it makes you uncomfortable.
- You can't handle that; it's hard.

- You're going to be overwhelmed if you do that.
- You're powerless.

Anxiety is, at its very root, demoralizing and self-defeating. It disrupts our capacity to be in control and assert ourselves effectively. It can temporarily deprive us of our ability to reason and make rational choices because it can be completely paralyzing. Anxiety doesn't prepare us to react appropriately; it actually discourages us from reacting—this is one of the ways in which it's different than fear. Aside from fear being based in logic and reality (my house is burning; my dog is lost), it also prepares us for the genuine fight-or-flight response that was programmed into our ancestors. Anxiety, on the other hand, confuses and distracts us. We aren't thinking clearly or rationally when anxiety strikes. We become immobilized, and we don't know why.

## Why Is Your Teen Anxious?

Great question—and one that I asked for years.

Breggin's own theory is that anxiety typically has prehistoric roots in childhood and throughout adolescence.[4] Your child may have been made initially anxious by separating parents, a bully at school, a teacher they found threatening, a dog that bit them while walking to school, child abuse (known or not known), repeated childhood moves, and so forth. The anxiety your teen is experiencing now has origins in events that probably occurred years earlier and has made an appearance due to one or more factors. It could be school stress, a breakup, a fight with a friend, or a sport-related concussion.

Something may have triggered anxiety that was already lurking within your teenager, and this is why it may be confusing for caregivers to put their finger on what's caused the sudden behavior change—it's often not linear. It can be extremely difficult to deduce the reason(s) behind it because events that eventually result in anxiety can be altogether unknown by caregivers and unrecalled by the teen—so the cause of your teen's anxiety may be completely unknown.

Anxiety can also be induced by life's common stressors and the inability to effectively deal with them—and then you factor in things like social media.

## Social Media

A 2017 *New York Times Magazine* article cites physical and intellectual insecurities, academic pressures, peer judgment on social media sites, and cyberbulling as factors contributing to the skyrocketing rates of chronic juvenile anxiety.[5]

Whether we like it or not, there is a correlation between social media and unhappiness. For years, I was one of the skeptics who responded to claims of social media being responsible for anxiety and depression.

But you know what? Studies don't lie. According to a large study of 750 American teenagers,

- 95 percent have a smartphone,
- 45 percent are online "almost constantly" in 2018 compared to 24 percent in 2014,[6] and
- 24 percent of teens surveyed said they thought social media had a negative impact, and the biggest reason was bullying/rumor spreading.[7]

Since 2011, the rates of anxiety and depression (among teenagers, especially) have skyrocketed, prompting a great deal of research on the topic. Results have consistently shown a steep spike in mood disorders in correlation with the popularity of social media.

Why is this?

Perhaps it's the sense that one is participating in social activities without having to leave the comfort of the bedroom. Social media is akin to a virtual living room, filled with a curated group of people whom we feel comfortable with and want to be associated with. Experiences are chosen and executed according to convenience and levels of ease. Essentially, kids are learning to handpick experiences that they know they will be comfortable with and people (typically other teenagers) they are content to be associated with. But this is not real life, and when confronted with genuine, real-life experiences, they clam up and back away. And why not? Why force yourself to be uncomfortable when you don't have to be?

This is a problem.

A study of more than 450 youth aged eleven to seventeen found that

97 percent of participants indicated that they used social media. Thirty-five percent of participants were categorized as poor sleepers. Forty-seven percent of participants were identified as anxious. Also (and here's the kicker), higher emotional investment in social media was *strongly* correlated with higher levels of anxiety.[8]

There's also the issue with comparison and judgment. When teens are consistently exposed to only the very best of what people can produce (we all tend to portray ourselves on social media in the best light possible—there are literally hundreds of apps for this), it creates a false sense of normalcy. The urge to compare ourselves to what we see online is overwhelming, and this can produce negative feelings of inadequacy and depression.

Results of a study conducted by the Royal Society for Public Health found that "Snapchat, Facebook, Twitter, and Instagram all led to increased feelings of depression, anxiety, poor body image, and loneliness."[9]

Maya, one of the teenagers we consulted with throughout the making of this book, told us that she will often take social media breaks, and some of her friends do, too. She conveyed that she will begin to feel very "low" and then delete her accounts, which actually makes her feel better. She finds that the less time she spends on her phone, the happier she is—yet she always goes back to her phone (and social media) eventually, even though she knows it makes her feel bad.

This is interesting.

What is it about social media and the need to feel hyperconnected?

## Smartphones

Social media aside, smartphones provide a distraction, which is enough to derail teens who are (unknowingly or not) looking for avoidance tactics. Scrolling through social media platforms and the incredible deluge of available apps or reading information online are easy ways to avoid actually talking to people or facing uncomfortable situations—something that everyone must get used to eventually if they truly want to prepare for the world beyond high school.

When friendship is conducted primarily online and mostly communicated via text message, teens are not experiencing most of the personal—and often intimidating—aspects of real communication. It's much easier to be tentative or coy when you're texting, so less is at stake. Teenagers aren't hearing or seeing the effects that their words are having on their conversation partner, and because the dialog isn't happening in real time, parties can take more time to consider a response. It's no surprise that teens often want their parents to "chill out" or "calm down"—we're speaking directly to them, and if they aren't used to doing the same with their peer groups, it's probably really overwhelming!

If teens aren't getting enough experience relating to people and having their needs met in person and in real time, many of them will grow up to become adults who are overly anxious about direct communication. And social negotiations only get riskier as people get older and begin navigating through complicated and grown-up situations like romantic relationships and employment.

It's incredibly easy to waste hours on a device capable of providing one with any information they desire in an instant, and today's teens are gluttons for instant gratification. In fact, the average teenager has an attention span of fewer than eight seconds—that's less than a goldfish.[10] "Twenty-five percent of teenagers report forgetting important details about their friends and family"[11] due to poor attention spans. Smartphones can't be helping this issue, and yet many children have one in their possession by the time they're seven or eight years of age.

Parents . . . we're setting our children up to be *goldfish.*

## When Anxiety Becomes a Problem

When ongoing and excessive fears begin to cause considerable distress or interference in everyday life, that's when you can safely assert that anxiety is taking over. It can prevent teens from engaging in age-appropriate activities or meeting expected developmental milestones. It is this combination of excessive anxiety *and* disruption in life that helps us understand that anxiety is no longer normal and has become a problem.

Common examples of excessive anxiety and distress include

- complaints of an upset stomach or other physical woes;
- seeking constant reassurance;
- becoming visibly upset before going to school, and often more difficulty returning to school after weekend breaks or school holidays;

- crying and tantrums when worried;
- lashing out or screaming; and
- trouble going to sleep or staying asleep.

Common examples of disruption include

- academic failure,
- keeping isolated or failing to join in and make friends,
- refusal to go on school field trips,
- resisting participation in new activities or trying new things, and
- school refusal.

If the scenarios above sound familiar (Cody exhibited 100 percent of these symptoms by grade twelve), that's when you know there's something more to your teen's behavior than simply "being a teen."

## Effects of Teen Anxiety on Society

Anxiety disorders can impact every aspect of a teenager's life but especially their social and educational functioning.[12] Because of this, the effects anxiety has on teenagers is not their burden to share alone. As a society, we're not blind to what's going on with the younger generation—it's having a remarkably negative impact on communities as a whole, and age groups who didn't grow up with the current pressures of education or stresses related to smartphone or social media overuse are baffled.

Kids won't get jobs, don't seem to understand the value in obtaining a driver's license, and can't be seen in the wild without holding a vape in one hand and a smartphone in the other. Actually, today's teens can't be seen in the wild at all—they seem not to know how to interact without handheld devices.

When I ask my kids to put down their phones and go play outside, they look genuinely confused.

"What do you mean? What would we do?"

I might respond, "Ride your bike. Or skateboard. Or climb a tree."

This is often followed by incredulous laughter because they think I'm joking. Why would someone want to climb a tree when there could be new posts on Instagram? And as these children become teens, the further removed they become from the idea of operating without having constant exposure to the global world. They actually become anxious at the idea of being without their phones or having to make small talk with someone they don't know, or not being able to use YouTube to be shown how to do something instead of figuring it out themselves.

No wonder today's teens don't want to get a job: without being in their self-made bubble of digital comfort, it sounds like . . . work!

Teens aren't motivated to work as young as they used to be, but once they do decide to work, the problem is the pay. That is, there's little of it. But in the era of 24/7 access to information, they've discovered that if they just commit *more* to social media, create a YouTube channel, and post regular videos of themselves online flipping bottles so that they land upright, they could possibly become millionaires without even leaving their bedrooms.

So what do they do? They post more and don't leave their bedrooms.

Teens are learning they are content conversing via their phones and that they don't need actual, real-life friends. They don't need jobs because they like sitting in their rooms, and don't need money for that. They don't have their driver's license because they don't need a car, and they're in their bedrooms. And then because minimum wage sucks, they do all of the above even more, convinced they can make more by simply hanging out online. YouTube star? Sure. Instagram influencer? Yes, please.

But what's all this online communication really doing for them?

Dr. Catherine Steiner-Adair, a clinical psychologist and author of *The Big Disconnect*,[13] writes, "There's no question kids are missing out on very critical social skills. In a way, texting and online communicating—it's not like it creates a nonverbal learning disability, but it puts everybody in a nonverbal disabled context, where body language, facial expression, and even the smallest kinds of vocal reactions are rendered invisible."

Without developing the necessary skills that enable them to properly and appropriately interpret body language, our teens are becoming emotionally confused and nervous in situations that require this type of interpretation.

## That Disconnect, Though

The word *disconnect* sounds simple and easy. Like pulling a wire from the back of an old radio or a cord from a power outlet. But the disconnect that we're talking about here (the one that is occurring between today's teens and their parents, teachers, extended families, and social networks) is serious and can lead to utter debilitation.

And you know what? I've had to learn this the hard way, but it usually begins with the caregiver.

In Dr. Vanessa Lapointe's book *Discipline without Damage,* she discusses (in depth) the trials of breeding a culture of disconnection. Children in our care need us to constantly reassure them that we aren't going anywhere; that they won't be left to fend for themselves. This constant seeking of us (the important adult figure in their lives) begins at birth and doesn't go away—certainly not before their brains are fully formed and mature.

"It is the mini-moments of disconnection, when parents are too focused on their own devices and screens, that dilute the parent-child relationship."[14]

In our current culture of disconnect, we appear to be more connected than ever before. Social media and smartphones make certain we can all be found at the drop of a hat and we can peer into the lives of others at any given time, just as others can to us—but it's fake. Real connection means actual conversation, the reading of body language, and the genuine interest in another person's feelings, emotions, health, and well-being.

Just because we're "connected" doesn't mean we're *experiencing* connection—and actual connection is what teenagers who are in the throes of chronic anxiety need from us more than anything else. If this doesn't inspire you to coax your child away from their smartphone, I don't know what will. I wish I'd done it long ago.

Aside from our kids having access to unlimited amounts of information at any time of day, what else can be blamed for their feelings of isolation, abandonment, entitlement, and uselessness?

## Going Old School

When you consider situations you found yourself in as an adolescent that ultimately helped you develop and grow into the adult you are now, what were they? I've asked myself this question extensively over the last few years, and here's what I've come up with (if you're a child of the eighties, perhaps you can relate): I babysat—a lot. I was given tasks and responsibilities that were mine to complete on a daily and weekly basis, and if I didn't, there were clear consequences that (gasp!) were actually implemented. I was required to drive when I turned sixteen. I was also expected to work as soon as it was legal to do so. I had a curfew. My parents checked my homework. If I received a bad grade, I was expected to ask for extra credit work to make up for it.

You know what all of this did for me? It *empowered* me. It gave me self-confidence and built up my self-esteem. It all taught me that I was capable, responsible, and dependent on myself.

Are we doing this stuff for our kids? Because I don't think we are, and I'm including myself in this statement. Somehow, today's parents feel overly guilty and responsible for their teen's failures. But instead of creating situations to help them build opportunities to achieve their own successes, we actually remove those possible circumstances by over-involving ourselves in an effort to ensure they don't become too uncomfortable.

This whole raising-confident-teens thing is backfiring, and it's our own faults. We're inadvertently depriving them of character-building experiences that are necessary for success in the adult world. Without those experiences to call upon, it's no wonder our teens are anxious.

## A Numbers Game

Statistics show that teenagers are more anxious than ever before. Here are some hard numbers taken from the National Institute of Mental Health and the Child Mind Institute:

- An estimated 30 percent of adolescents have anxiety disorders.[15]
- Of adolescents with any anxiety disorder, an estimated 8 percent have severe impairment.[16]
- The prevalence of any anxiety disorder among adolescents is higher for females (38 percent) than for males (26 percent).[17]
- The prevalence of any anxiety disorder is similar across age groups.[18]
- In the past ten years, there has been increasing recognition of anxiety in young people by health care providers, including a 17 percent increase in anxiety disorder diagnosis.[19]
- Yet anxiety symptoms are minimized or ignored. As little as 1 percent of youth with anxiety seek treatment in the year symptoms begin.[20]

- At some point, anxiety affects 30 percent of children and adolescents, yet 80 percent never get help.[21]
- Untreated anxiety disorders are linked to depression, school failure, and a twofold increase in risk for substance use disorder.[22]

## Chapter Summary

Here's what we can do to help our teens create healthier social habits:

- Curtail your own consumption of social media first—teach by example.
- Give your teen your full attention when they talk to you.
- Have an honest conversation with your teen about the dangers of social media.
- Educate them on the downside of comparison.
- Limit phone usage via phone plan and other means.
- Discuss acceptable hours and create a plan together.
- Develop ways to keep your teen busy with activities that don't involve their smartphones.
- Set up Wi-Fi access that is only made accessible to your child for a length of time per day that you're comfortable with.
- Educate yourself on the signs of increased anxiety.
- Actively try to create real connection with your teens on a regular basis (help them to differentiate between being connected and experiencing connection).
- Be involved in what your teen is interested in.
- Give your teen responsibilities to try to build self-esteem and confidence.
- Don't save them from falling or failing.

# 2

# SYMPTOMS AND TYPES OF ANXIETY

"Anxiety is the most common mental health disorder in the United States, affecting nearly one third of both adolescents and adults, according to the National Institute of Mental Health." —*The New York Times*[1]

TEENAGERS are notorious for being lazy, messy, unthoughtful, disrespectful, inarticulate (you may be familiar with what I like to call the "teenage grunt"), selfish, and generally scattered . . . so how do you know whether your teen is struggling with anxiety or just the average kid that drives his parents nuts?

As a caregiver, this is where it gets tricky. However, there is one giant red flag that can help you distinguish between the two: if your teen's behavior is crippling their own life (as opposed to simply making *yours* hard), it's probably anxiety related.

For example, teens can be rude and messy and late and unthoughtful and disrespectful. But if those behaviors are also coupled with the inability to leave the house or hold down a job for longer than a couple of weeks, or if they're losing friends, those can be warning signs of an anxious personality. Anxiety can make your teen feel removed from their own self (depersonalization) and/or removed from reality (derealization). Simply put, today's anxiety is "a response to insecurities and feelings of being overwhelmed without a recognizable cause."[2]

But it wasn't always this way; anxiety used to save our lives.

## Our Ancestors Had Great Reasons to Be Anxious

Despite all the negativity surrounding it, anxiety is in our DNA—and for a good reason. Back in the days of saber-toothed tigers, humans needed a specific biological response to a real threat that occurred on a regular basis: imminent death. When those threats reared their ugly heads, our ancestors' bodies responded brilliantly by immediately pushing a large amount of adrenaline through their bloodstreams. This adrenaline enabled them to initiate a fight-or-flight response that temporarily allowed them to run very fast, hear very well, and exhibit strength they didn't normally possess. Over time, the types of threats that our ancestors faced ebbed away, but fast-forward a couple hundred thousand years, and we still have that fight-or-flight response hardwired into our nervous systems—but we don't need it in the same way anymore.

Chronic anxiety is akin to experiencing a massive surge of adrenaline while lying in your warm and safe bed, trying to sleep. You start to sweat, your heart beats faster, your mind races, and your stomach is in knots. But why?

There's definitely no saber-toothed tiger hiding in your closet or under your covers.

## Emotional Symptoms of Anxiety

The following list is noncomprehensive but contains common emotional symptoms of anxiety. They include

- feeling overly and consistently cautious or nervous,
- actively avoiding anything unfamiliar,

- avoiding risks,
- worrying excessively about what one can't control,
- having a hard time keeping up,
- worrying about being left alone or possibly abandoned,
- feeling like everything may go wrong any second,
- wishing for better luck,
- finding it hard to focus,
- wanting or wishing others knew what was going on,
- feeling scared for no reason,
- wanting more security,
- being surprised by how well others cope when compared to yourself,
- developing rituals or obsessions, and
- feeling tempted to find an easy way out or a quick fix for problems.

When teens are consistently experiencing emotional symptoms like the ones above, they temporarily become a different person. They isolate themselves, their self-esteem plummets, and they feel stupid and slow. They're nervous about everything. They don't want to try anything new, and even things they're familiar with can become difficult.

As a result of these behavioral changes, the people around them—like their parents—respond in confusion. It's difficult to assess what's going on, and people become easily frustrated and irritated with their lack of involvement in regard to their own life. They notice this, which makes things even worse, and so the cycle of emotional disturbances perpetuates.

And then there are their physical symptoms:

## Physical Symptoms of Anxiety

Anxiety isn't just about emotional symptoms—there are often several telltale physical symptoms that accompany chronic anxiety. In fact, it's not uncommon for people who experience intense anxiety for the first time to think they're having a heart attack—it's scary!

Common physical symptoms may include the following:

- **Loss of appetite:** usually due to stomach distress
- **Weight loss:** a result of no appetite

- **Stomach pain:** typically caused by hunger needs not being met and mental stress
- **Constipation or diarrhea:** a product of digestive unbalance, due to chronic stress
- **Headaches and/or migraines:** sometimes a side effect of medication, but also a symptom of chronic stress
- **Physical and mental exhaustion:** caused by the brain and stomach not ceasing always to churn
- **Numbness in fingers and toes:** caused by rapid breathing/taking in insufficient oxygen
- **Rapid breathing:** a product of anxiety; the body's way of prepping for fight-or-flight
- **Having a dry mouth (known as *xerostomia*):** commonly caused by medication and/or dehydration

When teens experience physical symptoms of anxiety like the ones above, they are very frightened. They don't feel like themselves and, in fact, feel as if their body is completely foreign to them. They don't understand why they're sweating or why their hands and feet are going numb. They've never had headaches before, and now they experience them on a regular basis.

The confusion they experience because of their anxiety is, in turn, making them more anxious. Again—the awful cycle continues.

So the question becomes this (and it's a big one): What can we do to help our teens recognize the onset of anxiety (both emotional and physical symptoms) and shut them down before they perpetuate a cycle?

## Ways to Shut Down Anxiety Symptoms, Immediately

Here are ten tips to share with your teen on how to squash their anxiety:[3]

1. **Practice Breathing**

   When teens feel anxious, they tend to hold their breath and/or breathe in too rapidly or shallowly. To help overcome this, simply inhale slowly and deeply through your nose holding one nostril shut, hold your breath for eight to ten seconds, and then slowly exhale through your mouth. Switch nostrils, and do it over again.

This is called "alternate nostril breathing"; yogis call it *nadi shodhana pranayama*. Practice this technique throughout the day for about a minute at a time, or any time you are feeling anxious.

2. **Establish Contact**
   The more alone your teen feels, the more likely they will be to stress and worry. Try to get them out of the house; they could go for tea, go for a walk, or call a friend. Feeling connected with others reduces anxiety and suppresses symptoms.

   Remember that a lot to do with recovering is dependent on connection!

3. **Stay Present**
   Ask your teen to pay attention to what is happening now, not to the past or the future; to take one day, one hour, or even one minute at a time, if they have to. Try and get them to get in the habit of not thinking too far ahead, especially during times of chronic anxiety.

4. **Don't Be a Victim**
   Encourage your teen not to become a victim of their anxious circumstance. Some anxiety sufferers develop a sense of calm and comfort in their troubles, and most of this takes place on a subconscious level. If they're worried about their health, friends, or school, create an action plan to solve potential problems so they can feel more in control.

   Taking action reduces anxiety.

5. **Don't Take Things Personally**
   Chronic worry often stems from a lack of information. If your teen is feeling stressed because their friend hasn't texted back, explain that there could be extenuating circumstances impeding

them from looking at their phone. Maybe their friend is at a dentist appointment or driving.

Try to teach your child not to jump to conclusions about things and stress before stress is even necessary.

6. **Decrease Stimulation**

Teenagers who have a natural propensity to worry excessively usually need to decrease their stimulation. For example, suggest to your teen that they drive in silence, keep their cell phone ringer on vibrate, take a lunch break outside and with minimal people, or go for walks by themselves or with the dog.

Let your teen do whatever they need to do to decompress and calm their mind.

7. **Share the Worry**

Encourage your teen not to sit and worry alone. When we naturally talk about our worries, the toxicity starts to dissolve. Talking it through with others helps us find solutions and makes us realize that our concerns aren't as overwhelming as we'd thought. Be a good sounding board for their worries.

8. **Get Writing**

Suggest that your teen write their worries down on paper. Journaling can help them put them into perspective, as they may come to think of possible solutions to their problems. Some people like to make lists, a bullet journal, or keep a diary.

It's all about whatever works better for your teen.

9. **Let It Go**

Chronic worriers have a hard time letting go of control, as if intense worrying will fix the problem at hand. Instead, train your teen to let go by meditating or visualizing their worries melting away. They can imagine their worries and fears all located at their fingertips, and then visualize blowing them away like a dandelion gone to seed.

There's actually a name for this technique: it's called *grounding*.[4] Use whatever visualizations your teen may need to see and know that their worries are temporary.

**10. Get Moving on the Regular**

Exercising (especially cardio) when you're feeling anxious helps *a lot*. It helps to banish the anxiety from your body, and the more vigorous the exercise, the better the anxiety-riddled symptoms get cleared out.

When your teen is feeling anxious about something, it's easy to think that they will stay that way indefinitely. The tips in this chapter can help them restore a sense of balance and calm within so that they can begin to see things a bit more logically while searching for reasonable solutions to the problem(s) at hand. Shifting their emotionally hijacked brain away from the fight-or-flight response and into a clearer state of mind will enable them to realize that their problems are quite transient in the long run.

These coping mechanisms can really assist adolescents in putting their chronic worry into perspective and slow/stop both physical and emotional symptoms of anxiety.

### Cody on Symptoms of Anxiety

Anxiety, for those who haven't experienced it, feels like nothing else. It begins as an intense feeling of fear, and then once you realize what's happening, it becomes way worse because you know you can't stop it. When I think of feeling anxious, I think of overthinking, overheating, and generally feeling sick for no reason.

When I first began to feel anxiety, I became super introverted, not social, and found myself zoning out a lot. Once the anxiety became extreme, I started zoning out on my phone in my bed and ignoring hunger pains and the need for the bathroom.

Panic attacks started before school every day by grade twelve; I felt like I was going to throw up. I felt like there was no way anything was going to work out, hated it, and would think to myself, "What's the point in staying? I should just leave." And then I would.

Anxiety makes you think in the present only and never ahead; depression makes you think of the past. Either way, there was no future planning.

Meds helped a lot. Weed helped; it was a motivator. Pot costs money, so I had to make some, and then there would be something to do after my tasks were done. I think this is important. Not smoking weed but having something to motivate you to get up and do something. It could be anything.

What follows is a list of the most common types of anxiety disorders for teens, and their corresponding symptoms. It's important to keep in mind that it's not unusual for teens experiencing chronic anxiousness to have more than one type of anxiety disorder and for symptoms to overlap.

## Generalized Anxiety Disorder

A generalized anxiety disorder (GAD) is characterized by excessive worry or feelings of anxiousness concerning several events or activities during most days for at least a consecutive six months. Teenagers who are going through this type of mental health disorder can be extremely difficult to communicate with.

This is the type of anxiety that Cody displayed.

"Nearly seven million American adults—or 3.1% of the population—have generalized anxiety disorder."[5]

As with most anxiety disorders, a combination of stressful life experiences can play a role in developing this type—but research has found that brain biology is typically the main culprit in GAD. Teens that experience a generalized anxiety disorder have typically been found to possess abnormalities, including lower-than-normal levels of certain neurotransmitters, increased activity in the cortex, and decreased activity in the basal ganglia (a group of structures linked to the thalamus—located in the base of the brain—and involved in coordination of movement).[6]

This combination of abnormal brain functioning seems to create an overreaction to what would typically be normal levels of stress—kind of like an overactive fight-or-flight response.

"GAD affects 6.8 million adults, or 3.1% of the U.S. population, yet only 43.2% are receiving treatment. Women are twice as likely to be affected as men. GAD often co-occurs with major depression."[7]

Symptoms of a Generalized Anxiety Disorder:

- Excessive, persistent worry about multiple things over the course of at least six months
- Insomnia
- Chronic irritability
- Experiencing tension all the time
- Difficulty concentrating

## Social Anxiety Disorder

According to a 2018 report spearheaded by Child Mind Institute, the average age of onset for social anxiety disorder (SAD) is fourteen years old.[8] This is exactly the age Cody was when he started experiencing anxiety.

Teens that have a social phobia tend to experience a predictable and powerful uneasiness in social situations—especially those they don't choose to be part of. Events like family reunions, big holiday dinners, or even getting together with a neighboring family can make them extremely anxious. They usually fear scrutiny, judgment and, ultimately, humiliation.

Being in social environments like attending a wedding or somewhere they're expected to participate socially can easily bring on a panic attack, and because of this, the suffering individual will try anything to avoid these situations. This, of course, comes across as being antisocial and rude if the people around them aren't aware of what the sufferer is dealing with.

SAD affects fifteen million adults, or 6.8 percent of the US population, and is equally common among men and women, typically presenting around age fourteen. According to a survey conducted by the Anxiety and Depression Association of America, 36 percent of people with social anxiety disorder report experiencing symptoms for ten or more years before seeking help.[9] And that's the thing: teenagers won't typically seek help because they don't necessarily know that what they're experiencing is unusual. It's up to their families and people who know them well to notice what's going on and start the conversation.

By intervening as early as possible, the possibility for a faster recovery is greatly increased.

Symptoms of a Social Anxiety Disorder:

- Extreme self-consciousness, uneasiness, and fear of embarrassing oneself in social situations
- General avoidance of parties, get-togethers, and other social gatherings
- Displaying symptoms of being ill in most if not all social situations, such as sweating, shaking, stuttering, lack of eye contact, and paleness
- Panic attacks in (typically forced) social settings, like school dances or parties

It's important to note that there's a difference between being an introvert and being socially anxious. Introverts typically want to participate in social situations but have a limited amount of time they wish to do so. (Social gatherings eventually become overwhelming and energy draining.) Someone with a chronic social anxiety disorder will usually not attempt to put themselves in a social situation to begin with—the very thought of doing so can elicit panic.

Which brings us to the following.

## Panic Disorder

Panic disorder is typically characterized by panic attacks that occur without warning and clear reason—which is why it's not uncommon for people who experience a panic attack for the very first time to believe they're actually having a heart attack. In talking with a variety of doctors while writing this book, I was told that emergency room physicians diagnose patients who admit themselves thinking they're having a heart attack with a panic attack on a fairly regular basis. It happens all the time.

Panic disorders typically present in late adolescence and having an immediate family member with the same disorder can greatly increase your chance of developing one. Also, when panic disorders are found alongside a mood disorder (like depression), personality disorder, or alcoholism, this can increase the sufferer's risk of suicide.[10] This type of anxiety disorder affects about 2.5 percent of the population, which translates roughly to six million adults.[11]

Six *million*—and women are twice as likely to be affected as men.

Symptoms of a Panic Disorder:

- Constant worry about having panic attacks (because they're scary)
- Changing one's behavior to avoid panic attacks
- Chest pain, shortness of breath, profusive sweating, heart palpitations, experiencing a smothering or drowning sensation (similar symptoms to a heart attack)
- Sudden and intense fear about an imminent catastrophe occurring

## Obsessive-Compulsive Disorder

Most people recognize the phrase *obsessive-compulsive disorder* as its abbreviated version, OCD. Affecting about 1 percent of the population, this particular anxiety disorder is characterized by highly distressing thoughts and worries that occur repeatedly and involuntarily (obsessions) and the behaviors or rituals that one uses to deal with the intrusive, upsetting thoughts (compulsions).

Very common compulsions include counting and recounting, repeated handwashing, repetition of words, and exercising to an unhealthy extent. Although it's common to have obsessive-compulsive behaviors from time to time, it becomes an issue and warrants the anxious OCD label once the behavior repeatedly interferes with one's life in an overly negative capacity. For example, it's perfectly fine (and often encouraged) to double- or even triple-check answers on school exams for accuracy before submission, but if you can't hold down a job because you can't exit your vehicle without counting to one thousand first, this is a problem.

Teens with OCD will typically have obsessions and accompanied compulsions for more than an hour every day. These behaviors can interfere with their ability to attend school, work, and participate in regular family activities, such as having dinner together or even going for a walk.

Symptoms of OCD:

- Repeated, involuntary thoughts, urges, or feelings
- Frequent repetition of very specific rituals designed to make one feel better about the obsessions, including excessive handwashing, word repetition, and organizing
- Major distress if their regular rituals cannot be performed and/or completed

As with many other anxiety disorders, OCD has been found to be caused by alterations in neurotransmitters and variations in serotonin levels. Therefore, obsessive-compulsive disorder is typically treated with SSRIs—a type of commercial medication we'll discuss in the next chapter.

Interestingly, OCD has also been found to be an early symptom of a B12 deficiency.[12]

The average age of onset for OCD is nineteen, with 20 percent of cases occurring by age fourteen. One-third of affected adults first experience symptoms in childhood,[13] and looking back, Cody fell into this group.

Although not diagnosed with official obsessive compulsiveness, Cody used to have specific behaviors that he made himself complete before he could move on to another situation. These included removing the toilet paper roll and turning it around a certain way, replacing the roll, then doing it again and again. He used to have to say goodbye to visitors exactly three times before we closed the front door, and if he wasn't permitted to do this, he'd be very upset and cry. He also used to like to open and close doors a few times before finally locking them and walking away.

Most of these behaviors subsided by the time he turned five years old, but when he's overly stressed, even now, he'll return to mildly obsessive behaviors until he's feeling more comfortable.

## Substance-Induced Anxiety Disorder

This last type of anxiety disorder is one that I personally believe is important to include when discussing teenagers. Because many teens tend to experiment with drugs and alcohol, substance-induced anxiety disorder is something to definitely be aware of. It's also important to note that your own experiences with marijuana may be very different than your teen's, and cannabis should not be overlooked as a dangerous substance. These days, modified marijuana strains are readily accessible and a cause for concern because of their association with anxiety through prolonged use.

Booze, caffeine, nicotine, decongestants, over-the-counter diet aids, prescription ADHD meds (like Ritalin or Adderall), and cocaine can all produce symptoms of anxiety. I don't know about you, but I know without a doubt that my teen has used a handful of these substances to try to increase energy levels.

Does your teenager regularly play video games?

Energy drinks and caffeine pills are a huge part of the online gaming culture and can play a role in feelings of anxiousness.

Symptoms of Substance-Induced Anxiety Disorder:

- Nervousness and/or agitation
- Feelings of panic
- Corresponding high heart rates and blood pressure

Treatment for this type of anxiety disorder is relatively simple: remove the substance(s), treat any withdrawal symptoms, and the anxiety should eventually subside.[14] A whopping 20 percent of people who regularly take drugs of any kind—including caffeine and/or alcohol—have reported regular feelings of anxiety in combination with the substances they're ingesting.

## Ways to Support an Anxious Teen

Regardless of what type of anxiety your child may be dealing with, there are many ways in which you can assist them in growing and learning while they learn to cope with anxiety. Often, the way you respond to what your teen is going through will be observed by them and noted.

Here are some suggestions:

## Set Expectations

It's important that as a caregiver, you have the same expectations of your anxious teenager that you would of your other children (participate in family events, follow household rules, be respectful, do some chores). However, understand that the pace will need to be slower and there is a process involved in meeting these goals.

You can help your teen break down big tasks into smaller steps that they can accomplish. You can help role-play or act out possible ways your teen could handle a difficult situation, like interviewing for a job or taking a road test. Rehearsing stressful situations out loud makes kids more confident and more likely to try the strategy when they are alone.

## Cultivate Your Teen's Personal Strengths

It's also just as imperative to praise your child for facing challenges, even if it's just a smile and quiet pat on the back. And there's a lot you can do to help build your teen's competence. Search to find avenues where your teenager can show they're good at something. Also, be sure your teen has jobs around the house that nurture the perception that they're contributing to the family (this is more important than it sounds).

## Don't Hover

While tempting, it's best not to take over or do things for your teen. While this might help them feel better in the short term, the message your teen will ultimately receive is that you don't believe they can do it for themselves—which in turn will have your teenager start thinking they can't, either.

I made the mistake of doing this with Cody.

It's hard not to—you're desperate to help in any way you can, and you feel a huge responsibility for your child's struggles. That's normal. But by watching his every move and assisting him with things he should have been doing himself, I basically eliminated any type of learning experience he was going to have, and I undermined his ability to grow and build self-confidence. I gave him no room to make mistakes, and ironically, it was a huge error in judgment on my part.

I wish I'd have let him fail a little instead of constantly picking him up. By not allowing your teen to make mistakes and learn from them, you inevitably squelch important opportunities for growth and responsibility.

## Resist the Urge to Pass Along Your Own Fears

Try to keep your fears to yourself, and as best as you can, present a positive or at least impartial description of a situation. Let your teen know that it's safe to explore and experience while using common sense. It's not supportive to laugh or minimize your teenager's fears, but it is okay to show your child how to laugh at life's ironies and mistakes.

Learning to laugh at oneself is an important lesson, and the result can be stress-relieving for an adolescent with chronic anxiety.

## Work Together as Parents

It's important to work with your spouse or partner to have an agreed upon way of handling your teen's anxiety that you both feel comfortable with. It's imperative that one parent not be "too easy" because the other parent "demands too much."

This is very confusing for your child who doesn't know who or what to count on, and more often than not, your teen will begin to manipulate the situation in order to stay in their own comfort zone.

Work together!

## Implement Consequences

Although sometimes easy to do, try not to confuse anxiety with other types of inappropriate behavior. It's very important to set both expectations and have limits and consequences for unsuitable behavior. Parents who have reasonable expectations of their children and clear and consistent limits and consequences for their actions and choices along with love and acceptance tend to have the most competent, self-confident, and happy children.

This means not putting up with abuse from your teen. Teenagers (anybody, actually) who are drowning in anxiety are angry, and the result is often verbal or even physical abuse. This is not okay, is never deserved or warranted, and should not be tolerated.

Please remember that.

## Communicating with Your Teen about Anxiety

Why is it important to talk about anxiety?

Despite a lot of chatter these days surrounding the topic, teens may not recognize their anxiety for what it is. Instead, they may think there is something wrong with them. For example, adolescents may focus on the physical symptoms of anxiety, like extreme perspiration. Teens may think their bodies are gross and become self-conscious about body odor—and these thoughts might make them feel even more anxious and self-conscious.

The first step is to teach your child about anxiety and how to recognize it. Self-awareness is essential and necessary for working on developing a treatment plan. Communicating with your teenager about anxiety is difficult—I've been there. They're often very closed, defensive, and scared.

Here are the three main steps to take in order to start the conversation:

1. **Encourage Your Teen to Communicate about Worries and Fears**
   Start by describing a recent situation in which you observed some signs of anxiety in your teen, such as, "I've noticed you still haven't dropped off those resumes we printed off for you a couple of weeks ago." Then go on to tell your teen about some things you were scared of when you were the same age (especially if you shared the same types of fears) and ask if they have any similar worries or fears.

   This is called "coming alongside."

   You may have to prompt your teen by offering an example, such as, "I know some kids your age are kind of nervous about attending a job interview. Do you have that fear too?" Being specific can help your teen sort through confusing fears and feelings.

   When your teenager expresses anxiety or worry, offer reassurance by saying you believe (and perhaps understand) them, and that having those feelings is okay. Remember, your teen is bigger now, but will take cues from you—they're kids in adult bodies. Show acceptance of worried thoughts and anxious feelings.

2. **Stay Calm**

Remember: if you stay calm, it will help your teen stay calm, too. Here are three important points to communicate with your teen:

- Anxiety is normal. Everyone experiences anxiety at times. For example, it's normal to feel anxious when on a roller-coaster, or before a test. Some teens may appreciate some facts about how common anxiety problems are. For example, "Did you know that one in seven children under eighteen will suffer from a real problem with anxiety?"
- Anxiety itself is not dangerous. Though anxiety may feel very uncomfortable, it doesn't last long, it's temporary, and it will eventually decrease. Also, most people can't tell when someone is anxious (except those close to your teen such as yourself).
- Anxiety is responsive. It helps us prepare for real danger (such as a bear confronting us in the woods) or for performing at our best (for example, it helps us get ready for a big soccer game or public speech). When we experience anxiety, it triggers our fight-or-flight response and prepares our bodies to defend themselves. For instance, our heart beats faster to pump blood to our muscles so we have the energy to run or fight. When we freeze, we may not be noticed, allowing the danger to pass. This response is also called "anxious arousal."

Your teen may be interested to know that in reality, without normal levels of anxiety, humans would not have survived as a species.

3. **Help Your Teen Recognize Anxiety**

Find examples of how your teenager experiences anxiety in each of the three parts: emotional symptoms, physical symptoms, and avoidance behaviors. Write a list of each and talk about how each part is different and how they affect your teen in different ways. Remember that prompting is okay, but let your teen do the majority of the talking. While speaking out loud, we often hear ourselves say things we didn't even realize we were thinking about. Let your teen experience that; this is an example of how not to take away their opportunity for growth.

Finding other recovered teens to share their experience with your own child can also help. Hearing stories of recovery can be extremely uplifting, and one person I talked to even said it was the recovery stories that helped her the most.

Keep in mind that when the time comes for your teen to be the one who's coping better, they can further their own recovery by mentoring others who are struggling, too. We all need to learn from one another in order to heal—it's the way the world works. It's what ultimately unites us and inspires us to live more fully.

It may not seem like it now, but one day both you and your teenager will be able to feel empowered by this process, just as Cody and I do now. We still have a long way to go, but we've both learned so much, and the changes that Cody's been able to make are amazing.

## Chapter Summary

Here are some ways you can support your anxious teen:

- Pay attention to their feelings.
- Stay calm when your child becomes anxious about a situation or event.
- Recognize and praise small accomplishments.
- Don't punish mistakes or lack of progress.
- Be flexible while trying to maintain a normal routine.
- Modify expectations during stressful periods.
- Plan for transitions to take longer than what would typically be expected.
- Put your teen in touch with another teen who's recovered from anxiety.
- Have patience.

# 3

# THE TEENAGE BRAIN

> "The most important part of the human brain—the place where actions are weighed, situations judged, and decisions made—is right behind the forehead, in the frontal lobes. This is the last part of the brain to develop, and that is why you need to be your teens' frontal lobes until their brains are fully wired and hooked up and ready to go on their own."
>
> —Frances E. Jensen

THERE'S a reason every parent fears the teen years. The development that occurs in a teenage brain is incredibly extensive, and the process it takes to reach full development results in behavior that caregivers (and often teachers) typically dread. Defiance, extreme mood swings, illogical thinking, dangerous experimentation, and unusual sleeping habits that stem from impulsivity and poor judgment are among these actions.

But these predictable behaviors are not necessarily the teen's fault—they have to do with adolescent brain development and the timeline in which this development occurs.

## The Timeline

A child's brain is already mostly developed by around age six, but then there's a refining and polishing process that must occur in order to result in a fully functional adult brain. It's this process that results in what we recognize as "teen brain," and it's not finished molding itself by age nineteen—a person's brain will continue to develop well into their mid-twenties, which is why we are such different people at twenty years old than we are at thirty years of age.

Adolescence is a significant period of growth for the development of one's brain and mental processes, and this can explain why those who may be predisposed to anxiety often begin to recognize the emergence of that anxiousness in their teen years. And remember: this is all biological—we're not even factoring in environmental reasons for anxiety (yet).

The brain is flexible, and the main change that occurs during adolescence is a process that basically involves sloughing off unused portions of the brain to make room for further development of highly used portions. Unused connections in the thinking and processing part of your child's brain are "pruned" away, and at the same time, other connections are strengthened. This is the brain's way of becoming more efficient, based on the "use it or lose it" principle.[1] Interesting fact: this pruning is the reason childhood development experts suggest introducing your child to a variety of experiences and challenging them with things like music and learning a second language as soon as possible. If a child's exposure to these things is weak, portions of the brain that can be used for this type of learning can be sloughed if not used by the early to midteen years.

The process begins in the back of the brain, as the brain develops from back to front. The front part (the prefrontal cortex) is the portion of the brain responsible for your child's ability to plan and determine the consequences of his actions, solve problems, and control impulses. Not surprisingly, this part of the brain is modeled last, and changes within this section of the brain continue into early adulthood. Because the prefrontal cortex is still developing, teenagers are commonly more influenced than adults are by a part of the brain called the amygdala. The amygdala is associated with emotions, impulses, aggression, and instinctive behavior and can help drive their decisions and solve problems—which is why teens are often so emotional.

Sometimes your teenager's intellectual processes and behavior seems quite mature, but at other times your teen seems to behave or think illogically, impulsively, or emotionally. The back-to-front development of the brain explicates these shifts and changes: teens are working with brains that are still under construction.

As a caregiver, it's important to understand that teenagers are actually *incapable* of acting and reacting in emotionally appropriate ways and cannot make logical decisions in the same way adults can. As Lapointe writes in her book, "children are not just smaller versions of adults."[2] It's not their fault that they act or react strangely to certain stimuli or sometimes behave in ways that are confusing to us; it's part of healthy brain development.

Now factor in anxiety.

Boys and girls in later stages of adolescence (fifteen to eighteen years old) display greater stress-induced cortisol levels compared to individuals in late childhood or earlier stages of adolescence.[3] When you're stressed out as a teenager, it restricts your ability to make good decisions. Cortisol levels interfere with how the brain functions in regions that are still developing, which include the reward system and the prefrontal cortex.

Parents: *knowing this deficiency is half the battle.* By taking the time to think about the consequences of their actions and how these decisions line up with their long-term goals, teens can assist themselves in lowering their own stress levels—but we as caregivers need to teach them how and why to do this.

This is a point that Cody brings up later in the book. He conveys that anxiety-ridden teens tend to think in the future, but in ways that are hindering to progress. That is, they stress about bad things that might happen instead of thinking about their goals and dreams and if their decisions are in line with those things.

We need to help our kids practice the art of taking a moment to align themselves and their actions with what they ultimately want to obtain in the next few years—and we need to do this in a way that fosters excitement for the future and limits feelings of depression about the past.

## The Link between Anxiety and Depression

As you'll read in various ways throughout this book, anxiety and depression are closely linked. Researchers are discovering that because the two disorders share certain biological features such as particular chemical imbalances in the brain, they are often on playdates together in one way or another. One of the reasons psychologists highly recommend proper assessment before blindly prescribing a teen medication is for the purpose of knowing which of the two came into play first (which is key to successful treatment).

Is it more likely that your teen's anxiety produced depression, or did their depression result in anxiety?

Figuring out the underlying cause to mood disorders and anxiety (anxiety was once thrown in the mood disorder group but has since been distinguished from it)[4] is extremely helpful in creating treatment plans that will garner long-term success.

Generally, depression produces emotions such as hopelessness, despair, and anger. Energy levels are usually negligible, and depressed people often feel overwhelmed by the day-to-day tasks and personal relationships that are essential to everyday life.

This is different than anxiety.

Teens with anxiety disorder experience fear and/or panic in situations that most people would not. They may experience sudden panic or anxiety attacks without any recognized trigger and often live with a constant nagging worry or anxiousness.

Without treatment, anxiety and depression disorders can impact your teen's ability to work, maintain relationships, or even leave the house—which is exactly what transpired with Cody. And if you can't convince your teen to participate in a treatment process readily, the disorder eventually overwhelms them and creates total emotional paralysis. So how do we convince our teens to cooperate with what we believe would be helpful, when their underdeveloped brains can't compute with long-term objectives and goals?

This is tough, and this is where parents and caregivers need some education and direction. We need to help each other, which is why talking about our teens' anxiety disorders is so important. We need the support of each other to support our kids in return.

Here's what we know about the correlation between anxiety and depression:

- Social anxiety disorder has the highest correlation to depression in later years—twice that of other anxiety disorders and three times that of youth without anxiety.[5]

- When teens have depression alongside social anxiety, it is strongly associated with increased suicidal thoughts, self-harm incidents, and more depressive symptoms.[6]
- Social anxiety disorder with onset in adolescence leads to earlier symptoms of depression and poor social functioning as older teens and young adults.[7]

## Our Role as Caregivers

With all these changes taking place in your child's brain, it's important to remember that even though your teen may seem like they are more grown up and mature (yes, their feet are huge, and your clothes are probably being pillaged as you read this), teens still need to be protected and nurtured. Research shows that the incidence of poor mental health increases during the teenage years, and one popular theory is that this could be related to the fact that the developing brain is more vulnerable to stress factors than the adult brain.

But another theory makes sense, too: if a child's brain develops its emotional core first, and that child has not been made to feel consistently secure throughout this development process, the shaky foundation of emotional well-being affects how the rest of the brain grows. In other words, a child must feel consistently safe and secure to cultivate a teenage brain that is properly regulated.

Okay—did that just feel like a blow to you? Because when the idea was first introduced to me, I felt like I'd been slapped.

Didn't I provide my kid with a safe and secure childhood? Haven't I told him I love him every single day since before he was even born? The answer is yes, and it's probably a yes for you, too—but that's not the only kind of security that must be provided.

As caregivers, we must learn to let our anxious teens know that we can comprehend why they might be anxious and that they have a right to feel that way. That we're sorry, they're upset, and we want to help. We need to provide physical comfort and emotional support so we can teach them how to regulate their own emotions.

These amazing, developing brains need a consistent foundation of unconditional love and support—even when they're teenagers.

> "Children whose scripts about their caregivers suggest that the big person cannot always be counted on to respond to their needs are subsequently more susceptible to developing depression and anxiety than children whose scripts tell them that their big person can always be counted on. Children who feel secure will experience higher levels of positive mood and better coping strategies, as well as be more capable of regulating emotion."[8]
>
> —Dr. Vanessa Lapointe

Let's get this straight: I'm not blaming you. Without any experience and limited resources at the time, I forced my own son out of our home repeatedly—once for four months that extended over Christmas. I was actually convinced he would get tired of not having access to copious amounts of food and a hot shower and his comfortable bed. I honestly thought he'd choose to stop being moody and decide to move back in, get a job, and obtain his driver's license within a week or two.

Four months.

So, I'm not blaming you or pointing fingers—trust me. I'm simply trying to share what I've recently learned about parenting a teen with anxiety: patience, love, and the power of connection is imperative to assisting your child in improving their mental health.

## Common Setbacks

Because of the nature of anxiety, adolescents who chronically suffer from it tend to experience a few common setbacks. These are normal, and it's easy to understand why they develop. Anxiety can be absolutely debilitating, so milestones like obtaining a driver's license, scoring (and keeping) a job, and dating or cultivating new relationships, as well as events like graduating from high school or commencing college, can often be delayed.

It's okay—these things will most likely happen; it just may take a little longer while your child works through the anxiety and learns coping skills and mechanisms that will eventually help them get back on track.

### Driving

Driving is already nerve-racking when you're just beginning so factoring anxiety into the equation can make it completely impossible. When Cody was initially learning how to drive, he would often experience migraines and feel sick. Even when we hired a driving instructor to participate in the learning process, he'd come home after about forty-five minutes, instructor behind the wheel, and he'd look white and clammy and completely checked out.

There were a couple of factors that led to him feeling like this. One, the process invoked inevitable nervousness. Two, he'd get motion sick on tight turns and feel nauseated (most likely due to his prior twin concussions that we'll discuss in the chapter called "Head Injuries and Mental Health" on page 55).

Regardless, it took a while. While he obtained his learner's license (something mandatory in British Columbia) on his sixteenth birthday, he didn't move on to the next phase of the license until more than three years later. It was difficult for him to experience his friends completing the process much faster than he did, and this only lent to his feelings of inadequacy.

Have patience with your anxious teen when it comes to driving—they'll get there.

## Working

When we stop to consider the process involved in finding a job, we can quickly perceive how difficult this would be for an overly anxious teenager.

From the time Cody was legally eligible to work, he spent a good chunk of time thinking he didn't even *want* to work. (Why would people work? It sounds really hard!) And then he decided he did want a job but was too uncomfortable to "sell himself" to a potential employer. When he finally got around to feeling like he was up for this dreaded task, he went through the motions, but was obviously fearful, which interviewers probably perceived as lack of interest.

Bottom line? Getting a first job isn't typically easy for anyone, let alone a kid with anxiety.

The one job Cody did manage to snag around this time (he was eighteen) was with the help of a friend, and it lasted for almost two weeks before he had a huge panic attack one day and simply walked away. (Without giving his employer an explanation, he was understandably fired for this.) By nineteen years old, he wanted to be making his own money, he wanted to say he had a job and keep up with friends who already had jobs, but he was still having a difficult time actually making it happen.

As a parent, it was beyond frustrating and difficult not to compare myself and my first job experience to Cody's lack of all of it, but there was really nothing I could do. I couldn't force him to work, and I couldn't force anyone to hire him. It was a waiting game, and only Cody could speed things up or slow things down.

What I'm trying to convey is this: if you are frustrated at your teenager's lack of what we sometimes see as synonymous with growing up, I get you. I understand. But have patience, and know that with the correct tools and support, changes will happen.

It's all about those baby steps.

## Transitioning from High School to College

I write a lot more about school refusal and panic attacks associated with going to school later in the book in the chapter titled "Anxiety and Education" (page 63). But for now, know that getting oneself to school and being capable of absorbing information and participating properly is nearly impossible for an adolescent suffering from severe and chronic anxiety. Like I wrote in the introduction, Cody hasn't graduated yet. In the end, he was short by only four credits—the equivalent of one academic course. I believe this was the most damaging to Cody's self-esteem. Above everything else, feeling like a failure for not completing high school was awful for him.

I also believe that I may have unintentionally played a large role in this happening.

By the middle of his twelfth year, Cody was not on track to graduate, and the panic that ensued from that knowledge on my behalf did not help the situation. I helicoptered the hell out of my kid, and that only increased his stress and anxiety. I didn't understand. His teachers didn't understand. The school administrator didn't understand. Cody didn't even understand what was happening, but the pressure he felt from me and others to knock it off and pass his classes was in direct opposition to what he really needed: us to all acknowledge his struggle and support him in as many ways as possible—and that didn't happen.

Please learn from my mistake on this one: if your teen is taking a nose dive and his anxiety is through the roof, recognize that he needs support and gentle guidance and love. He probably doesn't need a tutor and a tighter curfew—he probably needs you to hug him and hear him and work with him.

## Dating and Relationships

This is another area of struggle for anxious teens, because, as we all know, relationships are hard. Dating is confusing. For a kid who's operating on high levels of anxiety on a daily basis, these things would only add to their repertoire of stress. They may not want to go there for a while, and that's okay.

Don't pressure your teen to make friends and/or date if they aren't ready or don't seem excited about it. They're working on their foundation of mental health and trust me, going to a movie with someone they don't know well is the last thing they probably want to do.

Have patience.

When we spoke to Maya about these issues, her response was simple: growing up is scary.

## Hormonally Speaking

As if anxiety wasn't enough, teens also have to go through a (not so) little thing called puberty. And here's something else I learned while my firstborn was a teenager: boys can be just as hormonal as girls.

*Seriously.* I had no idea!

But girls also menstruate, which comes with a whole other bag of fun things to be anxious about. Bleeding through your clothing. An aching back and stomach due to cramping. The idea of a boy you like seeing a tampon in your purse. The list goes on and on. If your teen who is suffering with chronic anxiety is female, then add those things to the list of what she could possibly be anxious about.

That being said, a colleague of mine recently brought up something to do with this that I wanted to include in this book. She told me that downloading and using a period tracker app on her phone helped her control her anxiety. She relayed that by tracking her period status, she would feel better about how she was feeling if it was around the time of her period because it meant she was feeling anxious for a reason—that it wasn't just all in her head.

She went on to convey that using mood-tracking apps in her teen and early adult years assisted her greatly in learning what to expect from herself at certain times during the month—she found her anxiety was actually organized and had its own rhythm!

So, if you have an anxious daughter, this might be something to think about: apps that track her monthly cycle so she can learn her rhythms and know what to expect. It's also relevant to write that women of any age can feel anxious during menstruation or the days leading up to it, not just teens.

Boys can also do this—they obviously wouldn't need a period tracker, but a mood tracker? That may be of help. (I suggest a few apps for this in the "Resources" section of this book on page 165.)

## Intrinsic versus Extrinsic Motivation

In other words, internal versus external. Because anxiety is not a choice and teens typically feel very powerless when it comes to controlling their symptoms, extrinsic motivation doesn't often work very well. For example, I used to beg Cody to get his driver's license, and I'd promise him a car (an old one, for beginners) as a reward if he did it.

Didn't work.

I also told him one time that I'd give him a hundred dollars to come upstairs (he'd been in his bedroom for days without interacting with me or his siblings), and again, to my total shock, he didn't take the bait.

Why do you think he wouldn't go for these rewards?

I'll tell you why: because they were promises for doing things he felt he didn't have actual control over, and when you have anxiety so badly you can't leave your bedroom, you can't just snap out of it and decide to complete a task you would have already completed if you could have. Also, he saw no actual reward by obtaining his license or being handed cash—what would that accomplish for him, really? In his mind, nothing.

He needed to be intrinsically motivated, that is, motivated from within. No reward from external sources. He needed to tell himself that he had to do something and believe he actually could and for a good reason—one that made sense to him. That something positive (or whatever he deemed as positive) would come of his action.

So when he decided he needed to try medication again, he did so without argument or delay because he motivated himself internally.

What I'm trying to say is this: If you're trying to motivate your teen by promising them rewards for their actions that *you* deem necessary and/or relevant, don't. They need to make decisions for themselves in order for those decisions to be deemed relevant. And when they do make those decisions, they'll be proud of themselves for making them, and their self-esteem and confidence will raise a notch.

When this happens, be sure to take the time to validate and acknowledge these small accomplishments, because although they might be small for you, they may be huge for your teen.

## Parenting Your Stressed-Out Teen

Stress and anxiety sometimes can feel like the same thing. Both are healthy in small doses when warranted, and both can cause similar symptoms. The difference is that stress doesn't typically persist the way anxiety does and doesn't cause the same level of debilitation. Also, there's usually an obvious reason for stress, whereas the source(s) of your teen's anxiety can be very confusing and frustrating to flesh out.

Teenage stresses can include alcohol and other drugs, high-risk behavior, experiences like starting a new school and peer pressure, or major life events like moving or the death of a loved one. But they can also include things like social media, family dynamics, and nutritional stress. And then it gets even more complicated for parents, because although that teen of yours needs nurturing, too much perceived protection and unwanted attention might not be good for your relationship either.

I'm not going to lie, parents. This is where it gets exhausting.

Instead, staying connected and involved in your teenager's life can help you to learn more about how they are coping with stress. It can also help you keep an open relationship with your child and ensure that they see you as someone to talk to—even about embarrassing or uncomfortable topics. Children are typically more likely to be open to parental guidance and monitoring during their teenage years if they've grown up in a supportive and nurturing home environment, so knowing this, here's a summary of everything I both researched while writing this book and experienced while parenting Cody:

**Do**

- Just be there. Teenagers need to know that they have a safe person to depend on, so work hard to intentionally cultivate a relationship in which you know you're providing that. For teens, this usually means simply existing and listening when they choose to share with you without judgment.
- Be available. Be around for things like rides, meals, chatter, driving lessons, homework questions, and whatever else they may need from you. As it is with most things in life, it's all about the little things when dealing with kids—and especially an anxious teen.
- Create casual conversation. Instead of asking pointed questions, try making small talk. It takes the pressure off and inspires real talk when your teen feels comfortable. Choose topics that are neutral, like the weather forecast, the family pet, or the neighbor's new car—something that doesn't require emotional investment.
- Ask them to participate and do things with you. (Keep doing it even when they only say no, because they'll notice when you stop.)
- Give them space. Your teen needs you, but they don't want you to hover and be annoying. They want to know that you're there when they need you to be around but trust them enough to let them be.
- Let them fall and fail and make mistakes. This is important for growth and development. When we constantly prevent them from failing or making mistakes, we inadvertently delay their growth. Teens learn from their actions, so if their actions are always overseen and closely monitored, it only delays them in their journey to growing up.
- Provide a safe, comfortable place for them to call home. It's easy to become frustrated and not understand what they're going through, but at a very basic level, they need to know they have a safe home base that is theirs. For teenagers with anxiety, this is everything. They need to know that they can always rely on

their caregivers for the essentials: food, shelter, and love. I truly believe I delayed Cody's ability to heal by not providing these things when the proverbial shit hit the fan.

**Don't**

- Underestimate your presence in their lives. Even when it seems like they don't notice you, they do.
- Take away their ability to be social. In the teenage stage in development, they learn so much from their peers, and they crave social interaction with friends. Their friends become more like their family at this age and removing their ability to be social as a form of punishment (especially for someone with anxiety) can be devastating and increase the likelihood of depression.
- Put too much pressure on your teen. There is so much pressure already and remember that they're dealing with that pressure with brains that are not fully developed.
- Helicopter parent. This is a tough one that I know all too well because teens and their choices can be scary—but this is no way to parent. It's exhausting for the caregiver, and it will ultimately push your teen away and create an environment of hostility and silence.

## Cody on Parenting an Anxious Kid

The most important thing you can do for your teenager who is living with anxiety every hour of every day is to give them space and patience. No pressure. Pressure makes anxiety way worse. Kids who are delayed on things like school or jobs or driving already know they're behind—they don't need to be reminded and pressured. We already feel shitty about it.

We know we're different, and we know our parents don't like it.

When the pressure on both sides gets really bad, some parents kick their kids out. This happened to me—my mom kicked me out for months. This only delayed me in learning to work through my anxiety and eventually feeling better. I was in a bad place, and I don't blame her for doing it . . . in truth, we both needed a break from each other because she was on me for everything, and I was being awful.

But it created delay.

My mom also didn't like me vaping, but vaping kind of trained me to breathe deeply and helped me to relax. In the grand scheme of things, it's better than doing something else to relax, like drinking.

I guess I wish parents would just understand that some things aren't as bad as others and to pick their battles better.

## Chapter Summary

As you've just read, the teenage brain is unique and constantly changing. It's working hard at deciding what information is important and what isn't; and those decisions are based on experiences. It's also biologically programmed to perform certain functions and develop in a specific way on a fairly predictable timeline.

Here are some ways to assist your teen during these challenging years:

- Understand how a teenage brain develops.
- Study up on stress and anxiety as it pertains to teenagers.
- Remember that your child's anxiety is not about you; it's about them.
- Be prepared for setbacks.
- Know the common reasons for teen stress and anxiety.
- Remember that high levels of extra hormones add to anxiety that's already present.
- Give your teen the opportunity to become intrinsically motivated.
- Be there for your teen.
- Don't hover or helicopter parent.
- Provide your teen with a safe, loving, understanding environment.

# 4

# GENETICS, STRESS, AND ANXIETY

"61% of teens with social anxiety were behaviorally inhibited at age two."[1]

GENES can have a lot to do with an individual developing an anxiety disorder. Studies suggest that having biological parents who have anxiety disorders greatly increases the odds of having a child who also develops an anxiety disorder. Even if the anxiety disorder itself has not been encoded into the genes, a teen's particular set of inherited genes may play a role in predisposing them to anxiety.[2]

It's also important to note that though it's totally possible that children may experience a predisposition to anxiety from the genes they inherit from their parents (just as they inherit alleles for certain hair and eye color), it's also common for children and teenagers to receive anxiety disorders from their parents via learned behavior.[3]

Here are some statistics regarding the correlation between heredity and anxiety:

- Girls are at greater risk for anxiety disorders, and this gender difference typically coincides with puberty.[4]
- Genetic risk factors play an important role in both panic disorder and generalized anxiety disorder.[5]
- Children of anxious parents are five times more likely to report or be diagnosed with an anxiety disorder than those with non-anxious parents.[6]
- Youth onset of social anxiety disorder is typically linked to a stressful event. Approximately half of all adults with social anxiety disorder can point to a specific and humiliating event that started it, while nearly one-third identified an acutely stressful event that likely played a role.[7]

## Know Your Neurotransmitters

Think of neurotransmitters as tiny (but incredibly important) brain chemical messengers. Although there are several different types of these messengers, the three we'll cover below are the ones you'll most likely hear (or have already heard) about in relation to anxiety:

### Serotonin

Serotonin has pain-relieving or numbing effects and controls sleep, appetite, and mood. Current research shows that serotonin plays a role in the control of mood, depression, and even suicide.

### Norepinephrine

Norepinephrine is a neurotransmitter that affects the cardiovascular system by tightening blood vessels and increasing blood pressure. It's also theorized to be involved in motivation and reward.

Low levels of this neurotransmitter have been closely linked to anxiety and depression.

### Dopamine

Dopamine is an important neurochemical necessary for movement and affects motivation. It also plays a critical role in the brain's reward center and is hypothesized to be strongly associated with substance abuse issues.

In postmortem examination studies, dopamine levels were proven to be significantly deficient in the brains of those who had a diagnosis of severe depression.[8]

Again, although these aren't the only neurotransmitters found in the human brain, they seem to be the ones more greatly associated with mood.

## The Genetic Component

Our genes are a definite and undeniable component to anxiety disorders. If you look at families, you'll often notice more than one person who is afflicted. The difference is how they may deal with their symptoms, though, so it may not be apparent at first glance—and there might not be another person who suffers at all.

Here is what's interesting: researchers have found that genes do play a role in whether a person is biologically programmed to experience mood disorders like anxiety and depression. But here's the cool part: these genes must be expressed by environmental triggers to be activated. In other words, an individual typically must have the genetic marker for anxiety *and* be exposed to situations in which those genes decide to emerge and begin to cause havoc with our mental state.

This explains why two biological siblings can have completely different experiences when it comes to mood. For example, my own sister has been fighting depression since a small child (diagnosed at age seven), and then went on to develop anxiety as an adult. I, on the other hand, have almost no frame of reference for what these afflictions would feel like because I can honestly say I've never experienced them. Short from feeling blue from time to time during major life changes such as divorce or exhaustion stemming from the routine of a new baby, I've never felt depressed.

This, by the way, has not helped when trying to understand my teen. Not understanding what he's going through or how he's feeling and why has been very difficult. It makes me wonder if it would have been less stressful (and if I could have been more helpful) to watch him go through what he did, if I'd been able to relate genuinely.

## Stress and Anxiety: The Not-So-Dynamic Duo

According to data collected by the American Psychological Association,[9] teen stress and anxiety levels can more than rival that of their adult caregivers.

Results of one survey show that not only do teens acknowledge that their stress and anxiety levels aren't healthy, they also severely underestimate the impact these chronic disorders have on their long-term mental and physical health.

For teens, the most commonly reported sources of stress are as follows:

- School (83 percent)
- Getting into a good college or deciding what to do after high school (69 percent)
- Financial concerns for their family (65 percent)

More than a third of teens taking part in the study reported lying awake at night, overeating or eating unhealthy foods, and skipping meals due to stress. Forty percent of teens reported feeling irritable or angry at any given time, 36 percent reported feeling nervous or anxious, the same percentage reported feeling fatigued or tired, and 31 percent reported feeling overwhelmed due to stress. More than one-quarter of teens during the course of the study admitted that they regularly snap at or are short with classmates or teammates when stressed. Just over half of teens said someone tells them they seem stressed at least once a month.[10]

## Signs and Symptoms of Stress

All teens experience some amount of stress, and some stress can even be healthy. Many teens, however, struggle with significant stress levels that interfere with learning, relationships, and other areas of functioning. Stress can manifest in different ways, and some symptoms of stress mimic normal teen behavior. To that end, stress can sneak up on teens.

It's important to know what to look for when it comes to teen stress, keeping in mind that kids are more likely to describe symptoms that are physical in nature rather than emotional:

- **Emotional changes:** your teen might appear agitated, anxious, and/or depressed. Pay attention to changes in behavior.
- **Physical changes:** teens under stress are likely to get sick more often and complain of headaches, stomach aches, and other aches and pains.

- **Behavioral changes:** look for changes in eating or sleeping habits, and avoidance of normal daily activities.
- **Cognitive changes:** you may observe your teen exhibiting decreased concentration, forgetfulness, and/or the appearance of carelessness.

## Environmental Triggers

All teens are unique, and stress can be triggered by a number of factors. The results of the Stress in America Survey (where many of the statistics we just went over originated from) show that there are some common sources of stress in the teen population. The best way to understand how your teen processes stress and where the stress stems from is to engage in open and honest communication about stress. It's important for parents to normalize the concept of stress and empower teens to utilize adaptive coping strategies.

Consider these potential sources of anxiety for teens:

### Academic Stress

From grades to test scores to applying to colleges, many teens experience higher than usual levels of school-related stress. Many teens worry about meeting academic demands, pleasing teachers and parents, and keeping up with their classmates. Poor time management skills or feeling overwhelmed by the amount of work can play into academic stress, as well.

### Social Stress

We all know that teens place a high value on their social lives. They spend the majority of their waking hours among their peers (whether physically or virtually) and finding and keeping their tribes can include increased levels of stress at times.

Bullying and subtle instances of relational aggression are clear sources of stress on teens, but learning to manage healthy conflict and work through romantic relationships are also not easy for them. Peer pressure is additional stress during the teen years. In an effort to establish and maintain friendships, teens can engage in behavior outside of their comfort zones to appease their peers, and as a result, sometimes disappoint their parents.

## Family Discord

Anything stressful that impacts the family can affect the teen, just as teen stress can impact caregivers. Unrealistic expectations, marital problems, strained sibling relationships (including sibling bullying), illness in the family, and financial stress on the family can all trigger a spike in teen stress.

## World Events

School shootings, acts of terrorism, and natural disasters worry parents, but they also trigger stress for teens. Teens are often privy to the twenty-four-hour news cycle, and hearing bits and pieces of scary news, both domestic and abroad, can leave teens wondering about their own safety and the safety of their loved ones.

In a recent article, psychiatrist Stephanie Eken says that today's teens "wonder about whether it's safe to go to a movie theater."[11] I don't remember feeling this way; do you?

## Traumatic Events

Death of a family member or friend, accidents, sickness, or enduring emotional or physical abuse can have a lasting impact on teen stress levels—especially when left undiscussed.

## Significant Life Changes

Like adults, teens experience stress due to significant life changes. Moving, starting a new school, and changes in the makeup of the family (including divorce and blended families) can trigger stress for teens. Not knowing how to cope with big changes is overwhelming and can be confusing!

To make it even more perplexing, what might be stressful for one teen may be completely benign for another. But any of the reasons on the list above could be reason enough for genetically predisposed anxiety to make an appearance suddenly—and this would be very confusing for the afflicted teen. The sudden anxious state of mind can certainly be anxiety provoking, itself!

## Training Your Teen to Expect the Unexpected

It's been said that the only predictable thing about life is that's it's unpredictable. Change is inevitable, even though many of us try very hard to avoid facing it. The thing is, there are tools one can collect and foster that help with navigating change and finding inspiration in it instead of fear.

Here are some ways to help your teen see change as an opportunity for growth:

### Evaluate the Level of Control

Sometimes it's easy to become fixated on events over which we have no power or people who may very well never change their actions or attitudes. But rather than focus on blaming others or moving the unmovable, resilient people set their sights on what they *can* control.

To help your teen evaluate their level of control over a situation, ask them what they can take responsibility for in their circumstance. When you look for opportunities to empower them and teach them to become self-empowered and work toward change that is possible, they'll be less likely to feel stuck in difficult situations.

### Practice Postloss Self-Care

Life's transitions will inevitably involve losses, such as a death, a big move, the loss of a job, or the unwanted (or wanted) end to an important relationship. Even positive transitions, like a graduation or a job change, can make your teen feel more than a little sad and/or fearful. This is normal, but for those suffering from anxiety, these situations can have a very negative impact if the right tools are not in place.

During times of tough transition, remind your teen not to push away any grief they may feel. Encourage them to acknowledge the loss and pay attention to what they've learned from the experience. Help them seek support and camaraderie among friends and family and encourage them to consider speaking with a counselor or another type of mental health professional if they feel they may need extra support.

It's imperative to work through emotions because by allowing oneself to feel and deal with them properly, one grows and learns. Life is filled with ups and downs, and the faster we can teach ourselves to process emotions we view as negative, the more adept we become at rolling with the punches.

A really good way to expose your teen to healthy coping is by modeling it yourself. By demonstrating appropriate coping and resiliency, you normalize the experience and share that you are managing the change or transition, too.

## Create Mindful, Intentional Thought Patterns

In times of change, it's easy for anyone's mind to cut corners. Your anxious teenager may tend to see everything in black or white or assume the worst will occur. But if you help them take the time to examine their thought patterns and assess how rational they are, they may find some space to direct their thinking toward resilience.

Learning to slow down one's mind by practicing relaxation techniques such as mindfulness, deep breathing, or yoga can help your teen feel more in control. They can also learn how to increase positive thoughts by taking the time to remind themselves about transitions and challenges they've successfully navigated in the past. Help them make a list of ways they have been resilient thus far in life and consider what traits and actions might be able to see them through current challenges.

By focusing on their strengths instead of weaknesses, they'll feel more empowered to meet what lies ahead. This is important because people who suffer from chronic anxiety feel that they're very much out of control. This lack of perceived control can be completely debilitating, so educating oneself on how to gain more control is crucial.

## Be in the Moment

While it's important to look to the past to find your strengths, sometimes you can feel too pulled into the future in times of change. When your teen worries and stresses about what the future will bring or what mistakes they might make, they forget to be in the present and observe what's happening around them.

To bring them back to the present, your teen needs to get in tune with their body and pay attention to how it responds to stress, then set aside time every day to relax, take some deep breaths, and bring their focus back to the present.

With a little practice, this becomes easier and easier and can ultimately be very empowering for teens.

## Prioritize

The most resilient people see change as an opportunity rather than something to fear. Life's transitions allow us to consider where our priorities lie. How do we really want to spend our time on earth? What's really important to us?

Where does your teen see themselves wasting their time and energy? With a clear sense of their goals and values, they will find their mind and body can be much more resilient when it comes to the stressors of change.

### Cody on Environmental Triggers

For someone with anxiety, anything that happens outside of the bubble of familiarity is stressful and scary. Things like starting a new job, operating in any new environment, and anything not familiar is hard to process.

A couple of years ago, our family took a trip to San Diego. I wanted to go, but being outside of my comfort zone for a week was super hard. We stayed in a house on the beach, but I never went swimming. I didn't even bring a swimsuit. I didn't do much with my family on that trip; I spent most of my time in the house.

Things that bothered me included unfamiliar food, the area, and going places that meant I had no way out. We went to a baseball game there, and the noise was overwhelming. We were visiting somewhere cool, but all I wanted to do was go home and crawl into bed.

## Chapter Summary

Here are a few exercises you and your teen can go through to gather knowledge about anxiety and increase mindfulness on the topic:

- Familiarize yourself (and your teen!) with signs of stress.
- Ask yourself if your teen's anxiety could be inherited or learned behavior.

- Provide coping techniques for your teen that they can implement when encountering something new and/or scary.
- Give lots of information about situations that may be stressful (for example, helping your teen prepare for a job interview by role-playing).
- Explain why self-awareness is important and how one can become more aware.
- Talk with your teen about possible environmental triggers.
- Train your teen to expect the unexpected.
- Model appropriate coping mechanisms and healthy ways to navigate change.

# 5

# HEAD INJURIES AND MENTAL HEALTH

> "Individuals with a history of traumatic brain injury have significantly higher occurrence for psychiatric disorders and suicide attempts in comparison with those without head injury."[1]

HEAD injuries are scary at any age, but when our kids sustain them, the experience is awful—and sometimes the effects aren't just temporary. If you do a little digging online, you'll find countless scholarly articles from about the early seventies onward about the effects of head injury and its relationship to declined mental health. The gist is that head injuries can permanently create a state of anxiety, depression, and mental fog that contribute to confusion.

Here's what we have to understand: being diagnosed with a head injury means the brain has been damaged.

Brain injuries typically fall under two main categories: internal and external. An internal brain injury might be an infection, tumor, or stroke. External brain injuries might include a blow or hit to the head, penetration of the skull, and concussion.

## What's a Concussion?

According to the Cleveland Clinic, "a concussion is a mild traumatic brain injury caused by a bump, jolt, or blow to the head. The sudden movement causes the brain to bounce around inside the skull. This leads to stretching and damaging of brain cells and chemical changes in the brain. A jolt to the body can also cause a concussion if the impact is strong enough to cause the head to forcefully jerk backward, forward, or to the side."[2]

Most medical professionals would classify a concussion as a mild brain injury because concussions are usually not life-threatening. Even so, the effects of a concussion can be serious because they cause a decrease in functioning, and as I've experienced in my own life, they can go on to mold and shape into other long-term health issues.

> "Nearly 3.8 million people in the United States suffer concussions every year. Researchers using an MRI technique that measures the integrity of the brain's white matter found unique white matter injury patterns in post-concussion patients who had depression or anxiety."
>
> —Radiological Society of North America[3]

Adolescents are at higher risk because of their developing brains. Vehicle accidents, falls, and sports injuries are common causes of concussions. Among teenagers, most concussions occur while riding a bike; being involved in car accidents; falling down (perhaps while drinking with friends); getting into fights; or when playing sports such as football, basketball, lacrosse, or soccer.

The most common symptom of a concussion is a headache. This is an especially serious symptom if the headache gets worse over time, which might mean that there is bleeding in the skull.

Other symptoms include the following:

- Nausea
- Dizziness
- Double or blurry vision
- Sensitivity to light and noise

- Fatigue or drowsiness
- Changes in sleep patterns
- Trouble comprehending and/or concentrating
- Depression and/or anxiety
- Irritability, nervousness, or sadness
- Seizures
- Not knowing people or places
- Unusual behavior

## Sports and Concussions

If you or your kids play sports, you're probably aware of the dangers of sustaining concussions. But how often have you heard about the relationship between concussions (especially repeated ones) and anxiety?

The relationship is *real.*

Although concussions have been given more serious thought of late than in the past, they still don't seem to be treated as seriously as they should. As I've found out along this path of educating myself about brain injury and its relationship to declining mental health, concussions can cause a whole lot more damage than people initially realize.

When Cody was fourteen and fifteen, he, unfortunately, experienced two concussions within a nine-month span of each other; both while playing hockey. This subsequently put a serious hold on sports for him, which inadvertently affected his perceived sense of self. He wasn't a hockey player anymore, and hockey was something that was building his confidence during a time in his life (adolescence) when confidence building is very important.

Now what?

## Concussions and Identity

Identifying with other people and various groups is the way we build our perception or script about who we are as individuals and how we fit into society at large. This begins at birth, but becomes especially important as teenagers, because who we identify with (and as) at this precarious age of intense growth typically goes on to define who we believe we are as we emerge into adulthood. When the perception of who we are is broken or shattered, it can be extremely confusing and even devastating.

Looking back, the period of time when Cody sustained those two concussions was the age everything began to take a downhill turn for him, and it wasn't until years later that we made this connection. A series of unfortunate decisions and events (including a gaming addiction, family life disturbances, and drug and alcohol experimentation) subsequently led Cody down a path that resulted in him developing rather severe anxiety.

## Identity

Your teenager's identity is firmly rooted in what they associate themselves with.

How a person identifies is ultimately who that person is, for all identity is ultimately in relationship to something else. An indigenous person identifies as "indigenous," for example, and that becomes part of that indigenous person's identity. The same person might identify themselves as male or female, a member of a particular religious group, a brother or sister, an employee, and so forth.

Even more personally, someone may identify as a loser, as someone who is helpless to influence the course of their own life, or as someone who needs to hate a particular religious group simply because that is what members of their own religious group are "supposed" to do. Though such personal beliefs may have no basis in reality, they are often taken at face value by the people who hold them. Such people act on their mistaken or irrational beliefs and end up creating problems for themselves.

Identity is not just what you know; it's also *how* you know because humans are not born with a set identity, as identity is something that develops over time. Young children have simple identities and see things in an overly simple, generally self-serving manner. As people grow older and wiser, they identify themselves with other people, places, and things in increasingly sophisticated ways and start to grow out of this initial selfishness.

Sometimes life events (such as head injuries) can interrupt this natural progression from selfishness to thoughtfulness, and people's identities stop growing. Such people may be chronologically adults but relate to others in the selfish manner characteristic of an adolescent. This personal identification can ultimately create difficulties for themselves and the people around them when their selfish expectations clash with their peers, who expect a more adult-like identity to be present.

We all know someone like this, right? Whose own identity is drastically different from what their peers perceive it to be? And when that person doesn't receive confirmation that their own identity is matched with what their peers observe it to be, this can create a lot of confusion for that person! Identity problems can cause people to have difficulty taking an appropriate perspective toward other important life tasks, creating a wide range of life problems.

Here are two common ways that identity problems can be present:

### Low Self-Esteem

Poor self-esteem occurs when you come to believe that you have little value or worth. This often occurs when key people in your life are critical toward you, or when you are a perfectionist and critical toward yourself. In either case, the tendency is to judge harshly, and ignore or play down the importance of real accomplishments, even when it makes no sense to act this way.

### Poor Self-Reliance

We all need to feel we possess a certain amount of control over our lives to allow us to get out of difficult situations or meet challenges we're expected to meet. When people believe they are helpless to alter negative situations they find themselves in, they tend to become depressed.

Though there are certainly many aspects of life that people can't control, there are a remarkable number of things that can be *influenced*. People who have poor self-reliance truly believe they are helpless to influence their fate, and will generally not seek to alter their lives—even when they are suffering.

## The Anxiety Link

There are hundreds of studies that have examined the relationship between concussions and teen anxiety. Here are a few conclusions they've come up with:

- A 2014 study that was presented at the Sports Concussion Conference in Chicago[4] concluded that teens who have experienced a concussion and are usually more sensitive to light and noise may also be more likely to have emotional responses—like anxiety. (These were Cody's symptoms, exactly: long-term sensitivity to light, noise, and anxiety.)

- According to the Centers for Disease Control and Prevention,[5] children and teens are more likely to get concussions and take longer to recover from them. But, just as symptoms of a concussion vary, so do recovery times.
- Researchers at the University of Kentucky[6] found thirty-seven teen athletes aged twelve to seventeen who had symptoms for an average of thirty-seven days after a concussion. Twenty-two of the patients in this group had emotional symptoms after the concussion, which included aggression, irritability, anxiety, depression, apathy, mood changes, and excessive emotional reactions.

Learning about the link between concussions and anxiety was shocking for me—if I had known earlier, I would have sought much more help for Cody in the weeks following the second concussion, especially. As it was, his treatment included filling out a questionnaire about how he felt and receiving massage therapy and active release on the muscles on the base of his skull. They didn't include counseling or therapy at all, and I, at the time, didn't have the knowledge or experience to ask for it on his behalf. Fast forward four years, and I was dealing with a teen who couldn't function in society—largely due to a complete loss of personal identity.

If you believe that this has happened to your teen, here are some ideas to help them navigate through what they've (hopefully) temporarily lost:

## Keep Your Teen Involved

After speaking with medical doctors who specialize in sports medicine and injury prevention and recovery, I've learned that one of the most important things we can do for our teens who are recovering from a concussion is to keep them involved with their sports teams. Send them to practices and games, even if it's just to watch. Get them involved with play strategy.

Do whatever it takes to make them feel like they're still participating and still part of the team—this helps to preserve their identities and assists in preventing the onset or severity of the anxiety that may be initiated or made worse by the concussion.

## Speak to a Specialist

It's so important to go over and above your doctor and seek the advice of a neurologist in the case of multiple or severe concussions. Although mild, concussions are still complex brain injuries and there are many things that can be done in the days and weeks to follow that will influence recovery.

### Cody's Concussion Experience

For me, there was a direct correlation between my concussions and the onset of my anxiety. I was fourteen and fifteen when they occurred, and I had mild feelings of anxiety (mostly around girls) before that, but then they heightened incredibly after. Initially, I was okay, but teachers were concerned because of my headaches. I liked school. I was really good at math, but after my second concussion, math became almost impossible. Teachers were sending me home to rest, and I started to like staying home.

My memory after both concussions was hazy for about two years. I couldn't remember simple things or situations. I forgot about everything and started feeling stupid.

This is when the anxiety really picked up speed.

I began overheating, was self-conscious about being lazy even though I'd been told to take it easy by doctors, massage therapists, my mom, and teachers. Friends wanted me to do stuff and became frustrated with me when I said I couldn't. I had to think extra hard about things.

Not being a hockey player anymore was hard, and the other thing I liked to do was play video games. My mom tried to take that away too because we were told it would make my concussion syndrome worse, but at the time, it would have been extreme.

Hockey and video games were the two things I liked to do.

I became obsessed with gaming, though, and started drinking energy drinks and snorting sugar and caffeine pills. Eventually, my mom took away my video games, and things took a turn for the worst. I became very angry. School is still very hard to talk about because I was good at it before my concussions, but I didn't graduate due to my lack of attendance.

I was (and still am—two years later) very angry at my teachers for not understanding.

## Chapter Summary

It's unfortunate, but concussions happen. While the injury itself may be inevitable or hard to avoid, there are definitely ways to help your teen recover faster and with fewer setbacks:

- Be sure to seek proper medical attention immediately after your teen sustains a concussion.
- Encourage your teen to take it easy, but be careful not to isolate them unintentionally.
- Help your teen to identify with another healthy group or activity.
- Provide access to both physical and emotional therapy, such as physiotherapy and regular appointments with a counselor experienced in adolescent concussion recovery.
- Communicate regularly with your child's teachers and keep his school informed of his well-being and progress.
- Keep a close eye on your child's mental health and recovery process.
- Be patient and encourage your teen to do the same.

# 6

⇄

# ANXIETY AND EDUCATION

"Anxiety is the most commonly diagnosed psychiatric disorder in children and adolescents. While there are many factors which result in anxious behaviors, school psychologists and other school staff can play an important role in helping young people to manage their anxiety and thrive."

—Child Mind Institute[1]

IT'S a rough time to be a high school teacher.

Aside from overflowing classrooms, underfunded programs, and half-staffed schools, teachers these days are dealing with kids glued to smartphones, fallout from social media participation, cyberbulling, and the subsequent increase in anxiety-ridden students.

And you know what? They're generally not supported.

These new mental health issues plaguing the average high school environment have not yet led to mainstream professional development to assist teaching kids that exhibit profound levels of anxiety—and according to studies, in a classroom bursting at the seams with an average of thirty students, there are definitely a few with anxiety disorders behind each door.

From a public health perspective, we need to advocate on behalf of our children for improving recognition (the earlier, the better) and increasing the rate of treatment of psychiatric disorders. An enormous amount of work needs to be done to promote improving recognition of the childhood anxiety disorders because high school students today have more anxiety symptoms and are twice as likely to see a mental health professional as teens in the 1980s. In fact, anxiety has surpassed depression as the top complaint among college students seeking mental health services (anxiety is the most frequent concern, followed by stress).

Because of the various types of anxiety that plague today's teens, it can be hard to spot in the classroom. Neurologist and former teacher Ken Schuster conveys that the commonality lies in the tendency for the anxiety to "lock up the brain," making school hard for anxious kids.[2]

A 2018 article published by Child Mind Institute reads, "While home and community settings can present difficulties for children, the school environment brings its own challenges. The development of social relationships, managing conflicts, problem solving, and understanding one's role in the larger social context are tasks presented to all children. Some are better at managing these tasks than others. Many children can feel anxious, ranging from mild to more severe clinical anxiety disorders. Mild anxiety may take the form of excessively worrying about a presentation or having minor somatic complaints. More severe forms of anxiety can manifest in the development of panic attacks in school or school refusal."[3]

The term *school refusal* only came across my desk while researching for this book, but the description is accurate. By the end of grade twelve, Cody literally refused to attend school. There was nothing I could do to get him out of bed, and admittedly, I was so scared for him that school became the least of my worries.

Let's explore this concept a little more.

## School Refusal

School refusal describes the disorder of a child (usually a teenager) who refuses to go to school on a regular basis or has problems staying in school.

They may complain of physical symptoms shortly before leaving for school or repeatedly ask to visit the school nurse. If they are permitted to stay home, the symptoms usually dissipate, only to reappear the next morning like clockwork.

Sometimes, a teen may even refuse to leave the home. (Like I said earlier, in Cody's case, it was his bedroom.)

In addition to not wanting to go to school, there are often many physical symptoms, including headaches, stomach aches, nausea, or diarrhea. In younger kids, tantrums, inflexibility, separation anxiety, avoidance, and defiance may be present, too. These are all common in the case of severe anxiety, and if it happens regularly, it should not be ignored, and the teenager should not be punished.

No one wants to be difficult or avoid friends at this age—there's almost always an underlying issue. In our case, that issue is anxiety.

Why?

Starting school, moving to a new house, and other stressful life events may trigger the onset of anxiety, and in turn, school refusal. Other reasons include the teen's fear that something will happen at home while they are in school, fear that they won't do well in school, or fear of another student.

But teens could develop serious educational or social problems if their fears and anxiety keep them away from school and friends for any length of time, so assistance is needed to get them back on their feet. Failing classes and alienating oneself from friends will only exacerbate a teen's anxiety in the long run.

Aside from refusing to attend school, students with an anxiety disorder may

- have a hard time concentrating in class or completing classwork;
- take prescription medication to help reduce anxiety;
- feel self-conscious and avoid certain situations;
- have physical symptoms, such as a racing heart, fast breathing, tense muscles, sweaty palms, a queasy stomach, and trembling hands or legs;
- miss class time due to problems coping at school; or
- need to talk with a school counselor or therapist.

## The Big Five

Here are the five most common reasons for high school stress, and ways in which you can assist your teen with navigating them:

1. **Fear of Failure**
   Kids who've struggled in school for many years often come to high school with a history of setbacks. Past failures can make the demands of high school feel even stronger.
   Your job is to remind your teenager about their strengths and about the strides they've already made. Talk about resilience and their ability to use past failures to move forward. You can also seek an expert's advice on how to overcome failure in school and explore tips to help them cope with test anxiety (which we'll cover later in the book).

2. **Competitive Academics and Increased Responsibilities**
   The academic demands traditionally increase with each year of high school. Even if kids have made great strides in middle school, they know the work will only get more challenging. At the same time, they're increasingly expected to self-advocate for what they need.
   Your job is to remind your teen of the support they have—both at school and at home. Encourage them to reach out to teachers for help. If they have an Individualized Education Plan (IEP), they can ask about having self-advocacy goals contained within this plan. You may want to look into tutoring options, help them find the right mix of classes and activities, and work with them to develop strong study habits and learn to slow down on homework.

3. **Increasing Social Pressures**
   Like I said earlier, social situations can also be a huge source of anxiety for teens. They usually feel intense pressure to fit in, be popular, and have lots of friends—whether these are real friends or virtual ones (friends made through social media

and/or through gaming). As teens become more independent, they may find themselves in new and possibly risky situations where they need to make tough choices.

You can help your teen by imagining possible dating hurdles they may face, along with common issues at parties (remember that these may be very different than the dating games we played when we were teens). You can also find ways to help them handle various school groups or cliques, and source out tips from experts on when it's important to let teens face the consequences of their actions.

### 4. Confusion about the Future

In high school, kids have to start thinking about what kind of career they want to pursue. They also have to eventually choose a path: university, work, vocational training, taking a gap year. If your child has an IEP, he'll go through a formal process to plan that transition—but that alone may not lessen the stress.

You can assure your child that feeling unsure or worried about the future is normal. Remind them that there are many ways for them to find success and happiness in life. You can also talk about different paths kids can take after high school and career options—including careers for kids who don't want to sit at a desk.

*Hint:* there are lots of them.

### 5. Concerns about College

Just thinking about attending college or university can be stressful for kids with learning and attention issues. But the process of getting there can create specific stressors. These include college entrance exams, filling out applications, and choosing a school.

Your job is to communicate with your teen about types of colleges and how they differ. If they are eligible, let them know that you'll help them find colleges that are a good fit. You can also try to give them a sense of control by discussing which might be better for them: college or trade school. Explain to them why it's important that they be the one to make the decision on whether or not to go to college and share realistic tips to help guide their choice.

Ultimately, you'll need to make sure the decision is theirs, and let them know you'll support them no matter what they decide.

## Test Anxiety

Test anxiety is not new and not uncommon. Although I've never really experienced it for myself, there are many, many people who have and currently do—and the people who are typically experiencing it the most are the ones writing a lot of tests: teenagers.

Here are five ways to help your teen combat test anxiety, prepare for their exams, and understand that setbacks happen and that it's okay:

### Keep an Eye on Their Schedule

It's one thing not to take enough time to study for a test; it's another not to have enough time. Feeling rushed can increase your teen's anxiety; help them leave enough room in their schedule to prepare comfortably.

Make it a habit to take a minute to glance over their schedule of classes and activities on a weekly basis, then talk about the amount of time they need to leave open for studying. You might consider suggesting they cut back on activities if that will give them space to breathe and to study without feeling like they're compromising something else.

Explain how keeping a relative balance can relieve stress.

### Avoid Procrastination

Although not uncommon for students, last-minute cramming for an exam is likely only to increase your child's anxiety, not lessen it. Part of the problem may be issues with organization and time management, two things that teens are not typically known to have mastered yet.

One way to avoid that is by helping them create a monthly calendar of tests. From there, help them set up a weekly schedule for review before each test or quiz. Review the test calendar at a set time each week and create the next week's study plan. Having a schedule mapped out and staying on top of it can help them feel more in control.

### Collect as Much Information as Possible

Some high schoolers become anxious when they don't know what to expect from the test. Is it multiple choice or short answer? Does it involve a skill they struggle with or a topic they find challenging?

Encourage your teen to ask their instructors for as much information as possible about tests ahead of time. Maybe they can take a practice test, or perhaps a study guide or last year's example might be helpful. Suggest that your teenager find out what type or combination of questions will be on the test or exam. Knowing what to expect can help them prepare and feel more confident going into it.

If they have trouble with integers, for instance, they may worry that this science test will involve chemistry. If they could practice in advance, it might reduce their anxiety.

By eliminating the element of surprise, your teen can better prepare.

### Provide Test Support If Necessary

Knowing that their specific needs are understood can help reduce your teen's test anxiety. If they have an IEP, make sure they know what it is and why they'll receive help. (Hint: they can apply for accommodations for college entrance exams, as well.)

You can also tell them that if his teachers forget about their accommodations, they should self-advocate and remind them.

### Prepare Your Teen for Setbacks

Even with good study habits, some students with learning and attention issues may not do well on tests. They may start dreading tests and become anxious over them because they're afraid of failing.

Try countering that fear by coming up with an action plan after a bad test grade. Acknowledge that you know what they tried and what didn't work well. Let them know you can talk about what might work better for next time.

## Common Myths about Teenage Anxiety

If you've never experienced anxiety yourself and didn't know much about it before your teen began to show signs and symptoms, then you may be confused about a few things—I know I was. Here are four common myths that seem to encourage misunderstandings about teenage anxiety (or anxiety of any kind that plagues anyone, actually):

## Myth #1: Having Anxiety Means That You're Mentally Weak

Let's get this straight: having anxiety has nothing to do with your strength of character. People with anxiety are some of the strongest, most likable, bravest people any of us will know. In fact, anxiety and courage almost always exist together. Courage doesn't mean you never get scared; if you're never fearful, there's never any need to be brave.

Having courage and being brave means that you're pushing right up against your edges of comfort and are making a push to move through them—and people with anxiety do it all the time.

## Myth #2: There's Always a Reason for Anxiety

Nope—sometimes anxiety drops in for absolutely no reason at all. It occurs because your brain thinks there might be danger, even when there is no danger to be found. This is one of the reasons why anxiety can be so frustrating: we can't always use logic to understand it.

It beats to its own drum.

## Myth #3: Anxiety Is Rare

In actuality, anxiety is very common.

On average, about one in five adolescents lives with anxiety. Without a doubt, someone you know or care about will also struggle with anxiety from time to time. Stats don't lie. They don't gossip, and they don't start rumors either, which is why they're so reliable.

Statistics are great like that.

## Myth #4: Anxiety Only Affects Certain Types of People

Everyone experiences anxiety on some level. *Everyone.* Anxiety exists on a spectrum; some people get it a lot, and some people get it a lot less, but we all experience anxiety on some level at some time in our lives via exams, job interviews, performances, relationships, whatever.

Sometimes it can happen for no reason at all.

Anxiety is a feeling, not a personality—it doesn't define you. Your brain is strong, healthy, and doing exactly what brains are meant to do. In fact, it's magnificent; it's just a little overprotective. It loves you like a favorite thing, and it wants to keep you safe. And alive.

## It's Definitely Anxiety . . . Right?

The first step in helping teenagers is to identify anxiety symptoms accurately, but anxiety is often mistaken for other disorders, resulting in ineffective treatment.

Common misdiagnoses include the following:

### Attention Deficit Disorder (ADD)

Youth who have difficulty concentrating in school but are not hyperactive may be diagnosed with ADD, while in reality, they're actually distracted by the internal worry and fear that come with an anxiety disorder.

### Learning Disorder(s)

When a teen starts doubting their abilities in a subject, anxiety can prevent them from learning or showing what they know. Sometimes this can be mistaken for a learning disorder when it's actually just anxiety.

### Depression

Teenagers who have been struggling with untreated anxiety for as long as a decade more often than not have a laundry list of things they can't do and/or haven't accomplished and are often unhappy because of their limited lifestyle.

That acute unhappiness can be commonly confused with clinical depression.

### Oppositional Defiant Disorder (ODD)

Teens who have acute anxiety may lash out when something triggers a fight-or-flight response. If the anxiety is undiagnosed, the aggression may be interpreted as a behavioral disorder like ODD.

### Psychosis

Older teenagers who have panic disorder or post-traumatic stress disorder (PTSD) sometimes experience depersonalization or derealization—a sense of detachment from the self or a feeling that the world is unreal. These symptoms may be misunderstood as a form of psychosis, resulting in a diagnosis of schizophrenia or some other psychotic disorder.

Sometimes we need to do our own investigative work when it comes to our teens' diagnoses. You know your kids better than anyone else. If a specialist declares your teen as having a specific disorder and you feel uncomfortable about it, or something just isn't sitting right with you, you need to trust your gut and find out if there could be more to it.

## Do Teens Feel Safe in Schools?

Aside from how we are educated to meet the needs of anxious kids and try to understand them, there's a current culture of fear that's circulating our schools, making it extremely difficult to ensure the safety of our kids.

Gun violence is a perfect example.

If you have a teen who is suffering from anxiety, school is already a difficult thing to push on them. But when the news reports almost weekly gun violence taking place at schools across the United States, how do you convince your kids that attending school is important and necessary?

How do we create a safe and supportive environment for our children whose mental health is already shaky?

A recent survey found that 57 percent of teens worry that a school shooting will happen in their own school. In 2018, when a journalist asked a Santa Fe High School student in Texas about the current state of gun violence in high schools, she echoed the feelings of traumatized students throughout the country by responding, "It's been happening everywhere. I've always kind of felt like eventually it was going to happen here, too."[4]

Aside from campaigning for stricter gun laws and homeschooling our teenagers, here are some tips on how to help kids feel safe:

### Maintain Structure and Routine at Home

Kids feel safe when their environment is organized and structured, and they know what's happening next. This is most important when they are feeling stressed or overwhelmed. It's not unlike when they were little, and bedtime consisted of dinner, a bath, a book, and a song before bed.

Maintaining mealtimes and bedtimes and keeping rules and limits consistent is important in helping kids feel safe. Routine makes us (adults) feel safe, too—predictably providing us with a sense of security.

## Minimize and Monitor Their Access to Media Violence

Research shows that by eighteen years old, the average American will have seen sixteen thousand simulated murders and two hundred thousand acts of violence via the media. This ultimately results in adolescents not being able to easily distinguish between what's real and what's just good acting—our brains become desensitized to what they're exposed to on a regular basis. Observing violence on television can leave youth feeling like their world is a scary place where things like that might happen at any moment.

Minimizing our children's access to violent images will help them feel safer and more secure and decrease the likelihood of them acting aggressively toward others, too.

## Reassure Them That People Are Looking out for Them and Protecting Them

While we can't guarantee our teens' safety, we can remind them how many people love them and are looking out for them. That list of people includes the entire family, school teachers and administration, their friends, the local police force, firemen, volunteer safety marshals, and the community of parents with kids in the school district as a whole.

There are a lot of people who have a vested interest in your child's safety and the safety of all the adolescents in your community.

Talk about this.

## Help Them Realize Their Own Strengths and Capabilities

When you see your child make a smart, safe choice, point it out to them! Let them know they're capable of making safe, smart choices and being aware of their surroundings. Teens will feel empowered to know that they have skills and inherent knowledge to stay safe in what they perceive to be an unsafe world.

### Recognize When They Need to Talk to Someone Other Than You

If your teenager is repeatedly expressing that they feel unsafe and/or unsettled or if these feelings are impacting their sleep or ability to learn at school, it's probably time to seek professional help.

You can ask your family doctor for a referral to a therapist, or simply look one up online who might be in your area.

## An Obvious Construct

Despite all the good intentions and knowledge that we currently have about school-aged anxiety, we still can't seem to break the barrier between sufferer and educator. One of the reasons for this might be that the North American education system has become detached.

(Yep—I'm using that word, again.)

Teachers and school facilitators (such as administration/counselors/support staff) aren't permitted to show affection toward their students (many would be extremely wary of giving an upset student a hug, even when they sense the student's need for physical connection), they can't reprimand their students (for fear of it being interpreted as inappropriate by either the student or the student's parents), and their hands are tied when it comes to offering simple advice.

There are reasons for all of us to be sensitive toward one another when it comes to unconditional acceptance, but we've somehow become *so* sensitive that we're afraid to do anything that may be construed as unsuitable or in some way offensive.

Unfortunately, this really limits the relationships between teens who are going through mental health challenges such as anxiety and their supposed mentors and instructors who could be assisting in a variety of ways but feel they can't due to possible chastising.

This brings up another issue: should schools not be hiring teachers who have an innate sensitivity and desire to assist their students with problems outside of trigonometry? Or is this simply not in the job description? And if it's not, should it be?

Our teens spend a minimum of thirty hours a week at school. That's a significant period of time to be surrounded by adults who aren't interested in their students' mental health, or, if they are, afraid to actually help for fear of misinterpretation of inappropriateness. What can we do at the community level to improve the relationships between students and teachers, administration, and support staff?

Because thirty hours a week is significant, guys. It's big.

## Chapter Summary

Here are some ways we can help our teens thrive in school in spite of their anxiety:

- Make sure your teen's high school is equipped to provide individual counseling with a school-employed mental health professional.
- Talk to the school's administration about possible classroom accommodations or modifications.
- Make use of special education services (individualized education plans, teaching assistants, special education instructors, online courses).
- Ask for a referral to external community mental health providers.
- Talk to your teen about school safety and how they're being protected.
- Praise your teen when they make safe and smart choices on their own.
- Be sure to provide your teen with therapy if they should need it.

# 7

# HELPING OR HINDERING?

GOOD intentions don't always pay off, and although I have no doubt that every parent out there has good intentions when it comes to dealing with their anxious teen, I'm also certain that there are many of us who are making some mistakes.

(It's okay; I made them, too.)

We want to see our teens succeed, and the panic that ensues after anxiety makes a consistent appearance and doesn't seem to be leaving anytime soon can definitely result in mismanagement of the situation.

We can start off by taking an analytical look at how we've been responding to our kids' chronic anxiety and deciding whether we think we're actually helping them develop skills to deal with their new reality or if we've been hindering their ability to do so—or both.

Adolescent anxiety can look very similar among teens, but how parents deal with their teen's anxiety can look vastly different depending on the family's parenting style and knowledge and experience on the subject of anxiety and mental health in general.

We all mean well, we all want healthy and happy children, and we all want to feel like we're doing our best to achieve those things. It's just that sometimes, although it comes from a place of love, we inadvertently make things worse or delay progress for our teens. Now that I'm out of the high-stress bubble I lived in for so long, I can look back and clearly see mistakes I made while desperately attempting to save my kid.

Here are five common mistakes good caregivers make when trying to help their kids cope with chronic anxiety:

## 1. Anxiety Accommodation

We feel bad because we don't want our teens to have to live with anxiety. We want to make it all go away, and so without a second thought, we do just that. For example:

- Our kids don't want to go to school, so we switch them to online courses.
- Our kids are afraid to practice driving, so we just drive them where they want to go.
- Our kids feel anxious about working, so we give them money to avoid having them feel left out of doing fun things with their friends.

Helping teens with chronic anxiety is a balancing act. You don't want to push them too hard, but you don't want to discourage them from taking chances and trying something new or intimidating. Sometimes it's tough to figure out where your parenting falls on the spectrum, but you can always ask yourself this question: Is my teen learning ways to help cope, or affixing themselves to a foundation of comfort where nothing changes?

As long as you can feel confident that you're being supportive while at the same time gently challenging your child to continue moving forward, you're doing a great job. By helping your teen develop healthy coping mechanisms, you're encouraging them to fight for their life back slowly. You're giving them skills to help them move forward, which is the direction to move in if they want to feel empowered.

## 2. Premature Fear-Facing

This mistake is the opposite of the issue above. Some parents are too enthusiastic when addressing teen anxiety and hate to see their teens suffer, so they force them to face their fears before they're ready.

The intention is good, but the method is bad.

For those of you who don't understand anxiety, it's easy to believe we can force our teens to face their fears and "get them over it." Unfortunately, teen anxiety doesn't work that way, and forcing teens to do things that they are not ready to do can backfire and result in major delays in general improvement.

Like I just said, handling teen anxiety is a balancing act.

Accommodating their fears is not helpful, but too much pushing can have a similar effect. They can both stop any progress from occurring, and this was what happened when I forced Cody to move out of the house. I truly thought he'd give up his "bad attitude" and come back with better behavior. This, of course, didn't work as I had envisioned at all.

Instead, try working with your teen to develop coping mechanisms that let them face small challenges. Small challenges add up to big results, and this is what I eventually (through trial and error) learned to do with my son.

## 3. Pressuring Your Teen to Hurry Up and "Fix the Problem"

Some parents want their kids to feel good again so badly that we try to fix the problem for them. They're the ones reading the books and participating in therapy. They're also the ones handholding their kids through the battle of teen anxiety, which isn't ultimately helpful. (This was also me—while writing this book, I learned that I was a very classic example of a parent who desperately wanted her child not to have anxiety. I get it. It's frustrating to see your teen move at a slower pace than you would like, and it's frustrating to understand the skills that they need to use, only to watch them not use them.)

Unfortunately, this is a battle you cannot fight for them, the same way I couldn't fight them for Cody. When you fight teen anxiety harder than your teen does, the following is almost guaranteed to occur: you inadvertently make them hide their anxiety (which is the opposite of what you want to do), and you make them feel overwhelmed. When this happens, many teens just give up.

Remember this: this is your teenager's battle, not yours. Be a supportive passenger, but remember that you're not the driver, and you never will be. Avoid sending your teen the implicit message that you should be managing their anxiety for them.

## 4. Mistaking Anxiety for Manipulation

Teenagers are master manipulators whose skill levels are beyond impressive. Let's just acknowledge that. I truly feel that if they could use that seemingly inherent talent for good, they could rule the world. (They'd probably get back at us for parenting them by sending us to bed early and making us eat our vegetables and we'd *love* it. But we wouldn't let them know—we're not new.)

Anyway, it's important to understand that anxiety is not the same as manipulation. It may seem similar in the beginning because let's face it: we're a little frightened and leery of our kids at this age. They can be pretty intimidating because they don't make sense to us—but we can't mistake good old teen manipulation for an anxiety disorder.

I've met many parents and caregivers who undoubtedly believe their teens use anxiety as an excuse, and at one point (again, in the early stages) I was one of them. But here's the thing: most teens are *humiliated* by their chronic anxiety and would do anything *not* to have this problem. When you view your teen's anxiety as intentional manipulation, you're going to parent them with discipline and annoyance—both of which will exacerbate the issue. (Trust me.) So the secret is to flesh out the difference between the two.

Here are my two rules of thumb:

If your teen starts the interaction that becomes overly emotional, they are probably manipulating you. Kids know their parents better than we know our kids, and they know how to push our buttons. They often learn where our sensitivities lie (guilt, abandonment, pity, rejection, inadequacy, intimidation, approval) and create a situation which elicits an emotional reaction from us based on those sensitivities. They might want something specific and try to get it from you by playing with your own strong emotions.

Example: You and your husband have just recently separated. Your son (who is living with you) wants to go out for a sleepover, but his grades have been dropping lately and he's being punished by not being permitted to hang out with his girlfriend past dinnertime. When he approaches you with his plan to go out and is reminded of this, he may get angry and tell you that just because you no longer have a partner to hang out with, doesn't mean he doesn't.

He's playing on your sensitivity to inadequacy. Amazing, right? This is manipulation.

Now, if the interaction that becomes overly emotional begins with *you* (if you approach your teen), then anxiety may be plaguing your child. Your teenager didn't want anything; they are simply responding to your words and actions.

Example: You've made dinner and call your daughter to the kitchen, but she doesn't come. You try calling her twice more and eventually walk to her room, irritated, to find her sitting on her bed. You ask her to please come join the family at the table and she starts to cry and says she's not hungry and asks why you keep trying to make her fat.

This is not manipulation, because she's not asking for anything—she has no angle. She has no reason to lash out and accuse you of this; her accusation is a direct link to her own self-esteem at that moment, and her comments are concerning and should be looked into more closely.

When you know what to look for, the signs of either manipulation *or* anxiety are there; but they're different and won't typically be presented together.

## 5. Anxiety Misperception

When it became apparent that Cody was suffering from anxiety, I racked my brain to try and remember what may have happened to cause it, or what situations transpired that I didn't know about. I had all types of fears and scenarios running through my head, including unknown physical and sexual abuse, gender identity issues, and more. I'd ask him about these things, and he would look at me like I'd grown a second head. His answer was always no—but I wasn't convinced. There must have been something terrible that triggered his suddenly anxious behavior. Right?

Wrong.

Here's a fact: teen anxiety is often irrational and not usually based on actual experiences that can be connected to their current state of mental health in a linear way. You don't have to solve the problem of why or drive yourself crazy looking for answers that are just not available. Your teen has anxiety because your teen has anxiety.

That's it.

So now that you know what not to do, what *should* you do? You can start by arming your teen with healthy coping mechanisms. Take them to a therapist that can help build these skills. Have them read a teen self-help book that will teach them methods or watch a parenting video to learn how to teach these types of skills yourself.

Whatever you do, give your teen tons of support and have lots of patience and love.

Here is a four-step plan you can follow to help your teen work toward developing better coping mechanisms to combat their anxiety:

1. Identify anxiety themes and triggers (certain situations/places/conditions that always seems to elevate their anxiety).
2. Teach coping mechanisms to face anxiety (exercises that can cultivate a sense of calm, like meditation/avoidance of toxic people that initiate worry).
3. Set up small challenges to help them face their fears (drive for just two minutes/come to the family reunion for just twenty minutes).
4. Repeat.

Place them in situations where they can practice mastering their anxiety by starting small and gradually building. By asking your teen to participate in their recovery or anxiety education actively and then creating situations in which they can take baby steps toward an achievable goal, you help to set them up for better self-confidence and eventually they'll feel ready to take control.

## Ten Things to Never Say to Your Anxious Teen

Again, we may have good intentions, but we forget that our perceptions about what our teens are going through may be very different than what they're actually experiencing, and our words can do some unintentional damage.

Here are some examples of what *not* to say to your anxious teen:

1. **Don't Worry**

   You simply can't wish away your child's anxiety by telling them not to worry—if they're exhibiting signs of anxiety, trust me, they're worried. Telling them not to worry implies that their worries are unreasonable or unacceptable.

   A better approach is to ask them to tell you more about their worries.

   Listen to what they say with understanding and acknowledge them. Say, "That does sound scary; I understand why you'd feel this way." Then pause and ask, "What's the worst thing that can happen in this situation?" Let them tell you what they think, nod your head, and agree.

   Then just wait.

   By working through their fears with them, they will eventually progress to the other side of the fear, knowing you're facing it with them. Here's an example:

   Teen: "I can't take my driver's test. I'm afraid."

   You: "I get that; driving is scary, and driving with a stranger beside you is intimidating! That's a totally legit way to feel about this."

   Pause.

   You: "What do you think is the worst thing that could happen?"

   Teen: "I fail my test or get in an accident."

   You, nodding: "Yes . . . those things could happen. But they may not happen, and you're totally capable of this. I'll be waiting right there for you when you get back from the test, and we can talk about what happened, after. If you don't want to try, no problem—I'm still here for you."

   Then wait. Let your teen think about it and decide after having communicated their fear with you. Accept their decision and move on. Regardless of whether the teenager in this scenario takes the test, a few things have happened: you affirmed and legitimized their fears, you've made yourself available to them and proven you can listen to them without offering advice or giving them an ultimatum, and they're now thinking about possibilities instead of just their fear, alone.

This is called "positive regard."

2. **It's No Big Deal**

Anxious children know that their worries are a big deal. Their worries can negatively affect peer relationships, family relationships, school performance, and other areas of functioning—and that's a big deal.

Try this instead: "I can see that you're feeling very anxious about this. Let's do some deep breathing together."

3. **You'll Be Fine**

Anyone who has ever experienced excessive anxiety or a panic attack knows that "fine" is not something that resonates with an anxious mind. When a child's anxious mind is racing, he doesn't feel anything close to "fine."

Reassure your teen with the phrase "I'm here to help you."

4. **There's Nothing to Fear**

Anxious kids actually have plenty to fear, such as judgment, peer rejection, failure, and the list goes on and on. You can't extinguish their anxiety with a quick phrase, but you can help ease their fears by opening the door to a conversation and talking through fears together, just as what was outlined in the previous example.

5. **You Just Need More Sleep**

One of the difficult parts of adolescent anxiety is that it makes getting to sleep (and staying asleep) difficult. A worried mind tends to race at night when the craziness of the day finally slows down and everything becomes quieter (which means their thoughts become louder). This isn't your teenager's fault.

Try doing a meditation app together before bed to help your teen (and you!) relax into sleep.

**6. I'll Do It for You**

Anxious teens want to confront their worries and be more independent, but anxious thoughts often get in the way. This can lead exasperated parents down the path of "fixing" and "doing," but that doesn't help your teenager build coping skills.

Use this positive phrase to help your teen work through an anxious moment: "I know you feel anxious, but I also know you can do this. I'm here to support you; I'm not leaving."

**7. It's Not Real**

Anxiety is *very* real and dismissing it as anything but will shame your anxious teen, increasing feelings of guilt. They already feel different and behind and unable to participate in basic experiences that other teens their own age are experiencing.

They don't need to be told that their struggle is not real—this will only lead to anger and resentment toward you.

**8. Hurry Up**

Anxious kids tend to move very, very, *very* slowly. While some get caught in the trap of perfectionism, others are burdened with feelings of regret when making decisions or the inability to make any decisions at all. Telling them to hurry up only increases feelings of guilt and helplessness.

Instead, ask a simple question to help your child move along, such as, "How can I help you?"

**9. Stop Focusing on the Anxiety**

Trust me, your teen would love to stop thinking anxious thoughts. The problem is that it's very difficult to interrupt the anxious thought cycle without proper supports in place.

Instead, try asking your teen what they're thinking about, and how you can help them feel better about it.

**10. I Can't Help You**

Parenting an anxious child is very difficult and often downright exhausting, but your teenager needs you to remain calm and hopeful in the face of their anxiety. If you express hopelessness, your child's anxiety will surely spike, because whether it seems like it or not, you are their anchor.

Try this phrase: "Let's brainstorm ways to help calm our minds right now."

It takes time and practice to learn to cope with anxiety. Your child doesn't mean to cling, repeatedly ask the same questions, or fall apart in the high school parking lot. Anxiety makes all of these things (and more) happen for many teens every single day.

Seek outside help to get your teenager the tools they need to learn to cope and do your best to respond with empathy and compassion when they come to you with their worries.

## Disciplining Your Anxious Teen

By their very nature, anxious kids tend to be sensitive, perfectionistic, and emotional. Because of this, discipline for anxious kids comes with its own unique challenges. But done positively, it can build your anxious teen and cement your relationship. Here's how:

### Discipline, Don't Punish

Discipline, as in "disciple." (As in, "to teach.") What you're aiming for are long-term results: the more they take on the lessons you provide them with as adolescents, the better prepared they'll be as adults.

Discipline is different than punishment. It's more important, more productive, and focuses on teaching rather than modifying behavior. Punishment will teach a behavior because of fear of consequences, whereas discipline will teach a behavior because that behavior comes to make sense. (This goes back to Dr. Lapointe's theory of disconnect. See page 9.)

It doesn't mean there won't be consequences; all of our choices have consequences, and that's an important lesson, but with positive discipline, the consequences make sense to your teen. For example, when your teen lies to you, it damages your trust in them. Focus on the lost trust and what that means for your relationship, not the actual lying.

Children and teens see the world a little differently than grown-ups, but the goal is to teach them about your world with love and respect. Taking on a behavior because that behavior makes sense is vastly different than taking on behavior in order to avoid the consequences. One leads them to correct their behavior, one forces them to hide the behavior.

Which way would you be most responsive to?

## Let the Value of the Lesson Be the Focus

Focus on the value to be taught, rather than the "wrongness" of the behavior. Respect? Kindness? Integrity? Honesty? Whatever it is, let this shape your response. For every rule, be clear about the value behind it. Have the conversation and let your teen know why it's important.

For example, if you've just found out that you've been lied to about homework, work out the value this violates. The biggest problem isn't the homework, but the lie—it violates the value of respect, honesty, and it violates trust. Explain this and talk about why the lie is worse than the behavior it's covering. When you have them on board with the values, they'll begin to write the rules themselves.

## Focus on Your Relationship

The better your relationship with your teen, the more effective your discipline will be. They want to make you happy, even if it doesn't always work out that way. Preserve the relationship by focusing on their *behavior*, not on them.

This is important for all adolescents, especially anxious ones. Anxious kids tend to be perfectionistic, and they need to know that even if you're not keen on their behavior, you still think they're amazing and that you love them no matter what. They'll be quick to see their transgressions, and you'll want to minimize the potential for shame.

## Keep Your Own Perfectionism in Check

Let them know when you get it wrong so they can see that everyone makes mistakes. Owning your own behavior is an important lesson to learn, and if your teen can see you model it, they're more likely to do it themselves.

Modeling your imperfections and your acceptance of those imperfections will help your child feel less pressure to be perfect. You might yell when you shouldn't, say the wrong thing, offer cereal for dinner one night, or forget to pick them up the day school ends early. It's going to happen, and it's okay because there's your opportunity to teach them a lesson that will stay with them for life: everybody gets it wrong sometimes, and that's okay—it's how we learn to do it better next time.

## Validate Emotions but Reject the Behavior

Youth feel what they feel because they do actually feel it. It's that simple. What they're feeling might not make sense to you, but to them, it makes perfect sense. The emotion is valid, but the way they're expressing it might not be. Teens are no different than we are—they need to feel heard.

If they don't, nothing you say will go in because they'll be too busy trying to figure out how to make you understand.

Make them accountable for their behavior, but let them know that you understand how they're feeling. Humans start to learn empathy from about a year old, and this happens by watching *you*. It's an important lesson for them moving forward that just because they feel something doesn't always mean that the right thing to do is to act on it. At the heart of emotional intelligence is being able to identify and respond appropriately to emotions in both yourself and others.

## Emotions Come First

As with any of us, times of high emotion are not the time for wisdom, lectures, explanations, or problem-solving. Don't try to make your point then; it's just not going to happen, and it'll make things worse. During periods of high emotion, the part of the brain that can hear rationality or logic is "offline," so they cognitively don't have the capacity to receive or engage in a rational conversation.

It works that way for all of us.

Instead, let your teen know that you're there, that you see them, and that you understand that they're upset. That doesn't mean you agree with them or support the way they're behaving, but it *does* mean that you can and want to support them when they're feeling fragile.

When teens are out of control, they literally can't control their brains.

(Back to teenage brain development, right?) They aren't doing it to be manipulative; they're doing it because there is something they need that they aren't getting and it's likely they don't even know what that is.

It might be attention, security, comfort, sleep. Whatever it is it will be valid, even if their way of going about it is unacceptable. If there needs to be a consequence, let it be for their behavior *while* they were upset, not for *being* upset.

Let them know all feelings are okay, but not all behaviors are.

## Manage Emotions

When you're setting or protecting a boundary, communicate your message as rationally as you can. This can take some Superman strength to pull off, but it's important. Stay with the message and don't bring in extraneous details. Speak in low tones so they have to be quiet and pay attention to hear you. Don't lecture, rant, or threaten to kick them out or cut off their phones.

By managing your own emotions, you can retain control of the situation and give your teen the impression that you can remain calm and levelheaded for them—something that is important to model.

## Choose Your Priorities Wisely

Nothing matters more to your kids than you do. They want to keep you happy, so they'll shape their behavior around your responses. If you make more of a big deal of messy rooms than you do about them being brave, they will inevitably move toward tidiness being the most important value.

We can't do everything, and neither can they: some things you'll just need to let go of. This will give them permission to let go of having to be perfect, too. There will be plenty of things that deserve high emotion, such as doing well at school, being kind, being helpful, and being brave. Save your high emotion for that and let the smaller things go. Spilling food on the floor never did anyone any harm.

Parents, pick your damn battles.

Also, keep in mind that anxious children usually expect a lot of themselves. Be alive to the possibility that you may be expecting too much or too little. If you overestimate their abilities, you'll add to their stress. They'll want to make you happy, and they'll push themselves to get there. On the other hand, if you underestimate their capacity, you'll undermine their confidence. If you believe they can, it will make it easier for them to believe they can. Make sure your expectations are age-appropriate, and be careful that your own anxiety doesn't weigh in.

## Emphasize Choice

Allow for choices within your routine. Give your teen the opportunity to have some control within the lines of the boundaries you've set. Teens need to learn how to make safe and smart choices, and they won't be able to practice doing those things if all the decisions are being made for them.

Mastering their own world leads to self-efficacy.

## Consistency Matters

Few things will stoke anxiety more in an anxious teenager than unpredictability. One of the ways anxious people relieve their anxiety is through control. This isn't done to be insensitive or bossy; it's done because of their great and very understandable need for predictability and safety.

The truth is that anxious adolescents don't need to control everything in order to feel safe, but they do need someone to take the lead, and as a caregiver, you're perfect for the job. They need to understand that they can trust you to be in control of their lives. To show them, be predictable and clear with boundaries and have confidence in protecting those boundaries. Predictability will increase their sense of safety and help minimize the likelihood of a response that's fueled by anxiety.

# Chapter Summary

This chapter was all about figuring out whether we're helping or hindering our teens' anxiety. Remember the following points:

- Periodically ask yourself if you're helping or hindering your teen.
- Try not to accommodate their anxiety.
- Let your child face their own fears, and don't push them to do so.
- Be supportive.

- Don't mistake anxiety for manipulation.
- Be aware of your own anxiety misperceptions.
- Study the ten things never to say to an anxious teen.
- Find ways to discipline your anxious teen appropriately.

# 8

# ANXIETY AND GUT HEALTH

IF you were born and raised in North America by parents who were also from the same area of the world (particularly Canada and the United States), you probably didn't grow up with the philosophy of the importance of treating your body as a whole.

In other words, the physical, emotional, and spiritual parts of ourselves are completely connected, and what affects one part will also affect the others. (You've heard the term "body, mind, and spirit"?) When we suffer physically, we also suffer emotionally and spiritually and vice versa.

Because of this, digestive issues are a prominent part of living with anxiety. In fact, stomach discomfort can be so normal that many people (and teenagers, especially) don't even realize that anxiety is affecting the way they digest food.

## Your Mind and Gut Communicate

Anxiety can play a huge role in decreasing the health of your digestive system, and what happens within the walls of your gut definitely correlates with brain health, too. Here are some ways in which chronic stress and anxiety can affect your digestive tract:

## Overwhelmed Nervous System

Contrary to popular belief, most changes that affect digestion don't start in your stomach—they actually begin in your brain.

The human brain has a limited amount of resources, and like we've already touched on, when your teen experiences anxiety, they're actually experiencing the overreaction of the fight-or-flight response that's designed to make it easier for them to escape danger. This response takes up a lot of the brain's resources, so their brain compensates by slowing down parts of the body that aren't as necessary to survival as others, such as the muscles involved in digestion, and circulation in the extremities (like fingers and toes).

Normally, since the fight-or-flight response is only supposed to be temporary, they would never notice that their digestion was altered. But because your teen's anxiety is a chronic issue, they're left with a digestive tract that's not working optimally.

## Neurotransmitter Variations

Similarly, the same neurotransmitters in your brain that affect your mood (like serotonin) also play a vital role in sending signals to the gut. While low serotonin can cause anxiety, anxiety can *also* cause low serotonin, which means that some of the chemical messengers that are normally traveling into your teen's body are very possibly being created at a lower rate, leading to digestion issues.

## Adrenaline Release

Another issue with poor digestion relates to adrenaline. During the fight-or-flight response, whether it be warranted or not, your body creates massive amounts of adrenaline to give it an extra boost in energy. In order to accomplish this, adrenaline needs to be created from your body's sugar stores. While this happens, your body starts processing nutrients at rates that aren't ideal.

This changes how your body processes nutrients, as well as affects your digestive health.

## Bacterial Growth/Immune System

Inside of your intestines are tons of bacteria—both good and bad. Good bacteria are designed to help you digest food and improve your overall health, but these bacteria need to be in the right balance in order to do their job properly. Good bacteria are constantly battling the bad bacteria, and in some cases, bad bacteria can win. Furthermore, good bacteria are only good when kept in check by other good bacteria.

When your teenager is experiencing high levels of chronic anxiety, their immune system is weakened and the bacterial balance inside of their intestines is subsequently affected. Those who experience chronic anxiety may have improperly balanced bacteria that is not digesting food correctly and ultimately causing digestion issues.

(This is where probiotics come in; more on that later.)

## Insomnia

A common problem that makes digestion worse is a lack of sleep. Sleep is an *absolutely crucial* part of digestion; it ensures that the body is at its peak energy level, so that food passes through at the right pace and your hormones and enzymes are recharged.

Anxiety can and does often make it harder to sleep. If your teenager is always sleep deprived, then they're creating physical stresses that ultimately contribute to an increase in digestive problems.

## Stomach Acid Gone Awry

Anxiety has also been linked to an increase or decrease in stomach acids. The effects of this are not entirely clear, but it's likely that instability in stomach acids creates problems digesting food and may even affect food once it goes into the intestines as a result of the higher or lower acid content.

As an example, people who have a tough time digesting heavy food (such as red meat and pasta) often have low stomach acid, which slows digestion and creates cramping, gas, constipation, and more. People with low stomach acid typically tend to do better on a vegetarian diet, because plant-based food is easier for our bodies to process.

## How Inadequate Digestion Can Contribute to Anxiety

Unfortunately, digestion issues can also contribute to further anxiety. Indigestion can create pain and discomfort, two issues that are known to increase symptoms of anxiety. Gas can lead to chest pains, and if you suffer from anxiety attacks, chest pains can often trigger them.

Any type of long-term discomfort has the potential to create or increase anxiety, so if your anxiety is causing indigestion and poor nutritional balance, there's a strong chance that the stress that poor digestion has on your body has long-term influences and consequences.

The correlation between anxiety and digestive issues makes sense when we consider how a human being is originally formed.

Our brain, spinal cord, and gut share a unique system called the enteric nervous system. Essentially, when humans are initially conceived and only consist of a mass of rapidly multiplying cells, our central nervous system and digestive system are one. Eventually, separation occurs, and each takes on its own important role in keeping us alive. *But*—they never completely lose that initial bond. This explains why our stomachs feel fluttery when we're nervous, or emotionally disturbing visual stimuli can make us vomit.

If the gut influences the brain and vice versa, wouldn't it make sense to feed ourselves nutrient-dense, kind foods that would promote optimally working digestive systems?

For example, eating greasy foods usually makes my stomach feel gross and gives me brain fog. I get tired after eating those foods, instead of obtaining energy—which is the purpose behind eating: to supply our cells with energy so they can multiply, repair, slough off, and so forth. However, when I eat things like raw vegetables, lean proteins, nuts, seeds, and beans my stomach feels good, my head clears, and I get an energy boost!

So let's apply this to teenagers:

## Teens and Nutrition

As with anything else, teens tend to lean toward instant gratification when it comes to food. I doubt very many of them consider the nutritional value of everything that goes into their mouths, and those that are more aware probably aren't as concerned as adults may be about the effects such foods tend to have on their bodies.

Because of this attitude, teenagers who experience anxiety only contribute to a malfunctioning brain by not keeping a meal schedule, pounding back mostly carbohydrates (carbo-loading), and consuming way too much sugar. Kids will especially do this when they're trying to increase their energy levels, which is what one does when anxious and depressed. For teens who have access to prescription medication, they will often seek "uppers" like Adderall to make them feel better. Fun fact: adolescents with anxiety and depression aren't typically as interested in consuming alcohol as they are in taking pills; alcohol is a depressant, and they're already low energy.

Throughout more intense periods of anxiousness, I've observed Cody with what appeared to be a nonexistent appetite, often not consuming any calories until midafternoon. At this point in the day, he feels sick because he hasn't eaten anything, but the anxiety he's experiencing is also present in his gut, so it becomes a hamster wheel of not wanting to eat while being hungry. If I were a betting person, I'd hypothesize he would take in about four hundred calories a day during these times.

At over six feet tall, there have been periods when he's been about 125 pounds, soaking wet.

You can't force a person to eat if they don't want to, which is why treating the anxiety is so imperative—how much more weight can one lose before they're just gone? At 125 pounds, his body mass index (BMI) sat at sixteen, which is very underweight. To achieve a normal BMI, he'd have to reach at least 145 pounds—which he achieved halfway through writing this book. (As I'm writing these words, he's over 150.)

Interestingly, as his journey into anxiety education and better health went on, his eating habits became much better. He began asking me to buy things like flax seeds and hemp hearts, presumably because he had begun to feel the difference those whole foods made to his stomach. He also became very fond of raw, local honey; Greek yogurt; kombucha; and dried fruit. He even began adding psyllium, collagen, protein powder, and almond milk to his smoothies!

These were all foods he didn't touch prior to commencing antianxiety medication.

He started eating raw carrots and cucumbers first thing in the morning and became very aware of his calorie intake; he tried to increase his calorie consumption by eating more and making the food he did eat matter. Not only did he gain some much-needed weight, he also inadvertently put himself on a more regular bathroom schedule. That regulation alone relieved some of the anxiety he was experiencing.

But not every teen makes this connection, and for many, stomach issues that arise or are made worse by chronic anxiety can add to the struggle.

## Irritable Bowel Syndrome (IBS)

IBS is a digestive disorder characterized by abdominal pain, cramping, bloating, gas, constipation, and diarrhea. A whopping 20 percent of American adults have been diagnosed with IBS, and women are more likely to experience symptoms (which usually begin in late adolescence or early adulthood).[1]

Although there is no known specific cause, some experts suggest people who suffer from IBS have a colon that is more sensitive and reactive to certain foods and stress. When I was doing research for my first book, *Happy Healthy Gut,* I found that everyone I had spoken to about this disorder could trace its commencement back to a stressful period in their lives—myself included.

Going back to the connection between the digestive system and the brain, people with IBS frequently suffer from anxiety and depression, which can worsen symptoms. The nervous system responds to stress, which makes many of us anxious and creates stomach issues. Evidence also suggests that the immune system (also responding to stress) plays a role.

IBS can definitely make one feel more anxious and depressed, and I know this firsthand. *Happy Healthy Gut* was written in response to my own digestive issues, and I've watched Cody fight with IBS both before his anxiety was first prompted, during his most anxious years, and then while the anxiety was on a steady decline.

Trust me—stomach issues and mental health disorders go together like two peas in a pod. Or peanut butter and jam. Or chocolate and nuts. (You get the idea.)

The bottom line is this, folks: the better you eat, the more you can help your anxiety. And the less anxious you are, the better your digestive system works. By explaining to your teen that helping one will also assist the other, this may induce healthier eating habits.

Feeling good is a fabulous motivator.

## Cody and Digestive Health Issues

Digestive issues are common but become exacerbated when combined with anxiety. In my own experience, it was not unusual to go days (sometimes over a week) without a bowel movement. Often when I was relaxed enough to feel like going to the bathroom, I'd be out with friends and would overthink it and wouldn't go, which made it way worse. The only time I felt truly relaxed was when I was with friends, and because we'd usually be somewhere like a park and it was the first time I'd moved around a lot for the last few days, my system would get going but I wouldn't be around a bathroom.

If I were feeling particularly anxious, I wouldn't leave my bed at all for the whole day, and even though I had to go to the bathroom, I wouldn't. The thought of leaving my room seemed so difficult that I ignored my body and waited for the urge to go away.

The other issue was my terrible eating schedule. I didn't eat at regular times, so that would throw my bathroom schedule off, too.

I guess what I'm trying to convey is that I've learned the importance of schedule and routine when it comes to eating and activities. And to listen to my body and go to the bathroom when I need to go, even if I don't want to and I'm comfortable not moving at the time.

Schedules have helped, but so has choosing my food wisely. I've discovered that raw vegetables, ground flax seed, and tons of water help. I definitely place way more importance on this aspect of my life, now. But it's hard to do when you're in the throes of bad anxiety.

You just don't care.

## Good Gut Food

When someone is malnourished, whatever the reason, you need to make every single calorie count—and the foods that contain those coveted calories must be easily digestible, absorbed, and used by the body. In other words, limiting crap food and providing nutritious sustenance is key.

Here is a list of foods that are really good for anxiety and ones that should probably be avoided:

Foods to Thrive:

- Fruit
- Vegetables
- Whole grains
- Plant-based proteins
- Beans
- Nuts
- Seeds
- Herbs
- Water and herbal tea

Foods to Avoid:

- Red meat
- Processed food
- Sugar
- Alcohol
- Caffeine

In Dr. Margaret Wehrenberg's book *The 10 Best Anxiety Busters*, her first "buster" is to avoid CATS—caffeine, alcohol, tobacco, and sugar. She insists that calming an anxious body and mind begins with changing the intake of these four substances and with limiting other unnecessary stimuli from one's surroundings.

## Probiotics

Probiotics are basically good bacteria and yeasts that live in our digestive systems. When someone is chronically stressed or anxious, probiotics will often diminish in numbers, which throws the good-to-bad-gut-bacteria ratio off balance.

When this occurs, digestive issues arise.

To help cultivate a better ratio of good-to-bad bacteria, you can give your teen probiotic supplements in capsule form. These guys can also be found in fermented foods like kombucha, good quality yogurts, kefir, sauerkraut, kimchi, and more.

If taking via capsule, I definitely recommend purchasing the kind that is stored in a refrigerator. Bacteria are living organisms and stay healthier for longer when kept in cool temperatures. The ones you find on the shelf probably aren't as effective as the cold ones in the fridge.

## Stress-Relieving Exercises

Because anxiety is closely related to poor gut health, there are several tried-and-true ways to calm the mind and stomach simultaneously:

### Conscious Breathing

Deep and mindful breathing can greatly improve your health in numerous ways:

- Allowing your body to create more energy, leading to less exhaustion
- Easier elimination of waste products and toxins, so that your metabolism can work more efficiently
- Better, more restful sleep
- Improved muscles, joints, and circulation of oxygen to all of your body
- Balanced and stable blood sugar levels

### Meditation

The digestive system is one of the biological processes most affected when the body is tense and anxious. When in stress mode, our body no longer focuses on everyday functioning, like digestion—everything becomes secondary to our body's fight-or-flight survival response.

This can wreak havoc on the gut, causing inflammation, acid reflux, ulcers, and even food allergies. By calming the mind and body, meditation takes us out of stress mode, allowing a deep level of relaxation so that everything improves on a massive scale, including digesting our food better.

Central to any meditation program, breathing deeply while focusing the mind can yield many great benefits. Blood oxygen levels and circulation are multiplied during meditation, which is of key importance to the digestive system (especially the stomach and intestines)—this makes digestion so much easier. On top of that, your digestive system's efficiency will build, providing not only immediate relief but also a long-term solution.

## Yoga

With a combination of deep breathing, stretches that target abdominal organs, and twists that massage and wring out stuck intestinal toxins, yoga relieves a wide range of digestive discomforts, like gas, bloating, and constipation.

This practice is also amazing for the whole body, so I would encourage your teen to give it a try. Join them! You could probably use the health benefits it provides, too.

## Abdominal Massage

Abdominal massage (which may sometimes be referred to as stomach massage) is a gentle, noninvasive treatment that produces relaxing and healing effects for some people. It's often used to treat digestion issues such as constipation and bloating.

## Aromatherapy

There are several essential oils that have been shown to help with upset stomach, calm spasms that disrupt normal motility, help alleviate nausea, provide calming support to the entire digestive system, and alleviate occasional gas and constipation. The rule of thumb for topical use is to mix one to two drops of essential oil with half a tablespoon of carrier oil (like coconut).

Here are some examples of what oils to use for improving gastrointestinal function:

- Fennel, ginger, and cardamom to induce bowel movements: gently rub one to three drops clockwise over the abdomen.
- Tarragon and patchouli are antispasmodic for normal bowel function: apply a few drops over entire abdomen and massage gently in a clockwise motion.
- Lemon and peppermint to help normalize acid balance: drink one cup of water mixed with one drop of either essential oil.
- Peppermint, ginger, lavender, basil, and anise for general stomach upset: drink one cup of water mixed with one drop of any oil *or* apply one to three drops directly over the abdomen in a gentle clockwise massage.
- Ginger, peppermint, and fennel for occasional gas: drink one cup of water mixed with one drop of any oil *or* apply one to three drops directly over the abdomen in a gentle clockwise massage.
- Clove and lemongrass to control overgrowth of unwanted sugars and yeasts that may take up residence in your digestive tract: place one drop of each into an empty capsule and take with food.

Please be sure your teen is not sensitive to any of these oils before allowing them to ingest them. They are all gentle oils with no known side effects, but it doesn't hurt to be careful. If you have any doubts and want more information, I suggest contacting an herbalist or naturopath.

## Chapter Summary

There are several ways to help your teen's digestive system when overwhelmed with anxiety:

- Make sure your teen is eating regularly. We could all benefit from adhering to a fixed food schedule, but this is especially important for people whose bodies are out of whack—it provides routine and helps to solidify an internal schedule. Create a regular eating schedule for your teen, and make sure they stick to it.

- Remember that your gut and brain are so closely connected that you can actually fool your brain into developing a reliable circadian rhythm by adopting a solid food intake timetable.
- Don't obsess, and don't let your child obsess, either. While a regular routine is definitely a good idea and highly recommended, nothing crazy will happen if your teen slips a little with this. If a meal is missed, life goes on. Just try and model good eating habits for your child, and they will take notice. Don't be on them for slipping here and there.
- Encourage your teenager to notice which foods don't work well with their body and eliminate them.
- Talk to your teen about the relationship between their digestive system and their brain and encourage them to pay attention to how one part of their body affects another.
- Consider stocking up on the good stuff and offering your teen primarily good gut foods. This isn't a suggestion to stop providing foods that your teen loves (you need an anxious teen to take in calories), but try to keep a variety of fruit, vegetables, whole grains, and other whole foods in your home.
- Add probiotics to your teen's diet. Probiotics are great for fabulous gut health, and I can guarantee that anyone experiencing chronically high levels of anxiety is depleted on these nutrients. Simply purchasing good quality probiotics in pill form and asking your teen to take one each day with food can make a huge difference to their overall gut health.
- Bring on the exercise. Introducing antistress exercises to your teen's daily routine can help their brain and gut to be better regulated. There are tons of studies done on the positive effects of exercise and brain health, so this method of assistance shouldn't be ignored or undervalued.
- Get your teen moving. Some ideas include the following:
    - Go for walks with them.
    - Provide them with a gym membership and encourage them to use it.

- Introduce them to yoga.
- Start hiking with the whole family every weekend.
- Ask them to take on the responsibility of walking the family dog.
- Find out if they'd be into participating in low-impact sports that are not necessarily team-based, such as golf, tennis, or swim lessons.

# 9

# NATURAL WAYS TO HELP YOUR TEEN COPE

"The need to find effective natural coping mechanisms for anxiety is greater than ever. A natural remedy for anxiety comes without the fear of dependence, and most antianxiety supplements also don't cause harmful side effects. In fact, many natural cures for anxiety are known to have other positive attributes as well."[1]

As caregivers, being equipped with the tools necessary to assist your child in making healthy decisions when it comes to coping with anxiety is imperative.

Why?

Because the coping skills we implement as teens will typically become our go-to mechanisms as adults. For example, most healthy grown-ups seem to understand the correlation between moving our bodies and stress relief, but teenagers rarely make that same connection on their own. Teens are all about instant gratification, achieving quick results, and anything to do with a selfish outcome. Therefore, many teens prefer to self-medicate to eradicate feelings of anxiety with alcohol and drugs rather than choose healthier options that require more discipline and self-awareness.

It's so important to educate our teens on the topic of substance abuse versus exercise and other healthy methods of self-care because it will ultimately determine how they respond to stressful situations in adulthood: the teen who temporarily absolves their anxiety with street meds is more likely to turn to alcohol as an adult. In comparison, teens who learn to work out stress and feelings of discomfort with exercise will most likely continue to use physical activity as a tool throughout the rest of their lives.

Here are some healthy, natural ways to help your teen cope with chronic anxiety:

## Cognitive Behavioral Therapy

Cognitive behavioral therapy (CBT) is the most widely-used therapy for anxiety disorders. Research has shown it to be effective in the treatment of panic disorder, phobias, social anxiety disorder, generalized anxiety disorder, and many other conditions.[2] This type of therapy addresses negative patterns and distortions in the way we perceive our surrounding environment and ourselves.

As the name suggests, this involves two main components:

1. Cognitive therapy works on how negative thoughts or cognitions contribute to anxiety.
2. Behavior therapy observes how one behaves and *reacts* in situations that trigger anxiety.

The basic idea behind CBT is that our thoughts—not external events—affect the way we feel. Basically, it's not the situation you're in that determines how you feel, but your *perception* of the situation. The same event can lead to completely different emotions in different people—it all depends on our individual expectations, attitudes, and beliefs.

For people with anxiety disorders, negative ways of thinking fuel the negative emotions of anxiety and fear. The goal of cognitive behavioral therapy for treatment of anxiety is to identify and change these negative thoughts and beliefs: if you alter the way you think, you can change the way you feel—perception is everything.

Here's a personal example for you. About a year before this book was an idea, I approached Cody in his bedroom and said the following words: "Cody, you're not going to school, you're not working, and you're not driving. What's the plan?"

He heard, "You'll never amount to anything."

He maintained that I said these words until I gave up days later and just apologized to him for doing so. And when I did, his faced cleared, and he genuinely thanked me for saying "sorry." He honestly heard me state that awful, demeaning sentence.

I would never say that (of course) and was confused about this until Dr. Carla Dassinger (that lovely friend of mine who happens to be a clinical psychologist), explained it to me. She told me that he *did* hear those words because they confirmed his core belief: at that moment, he truly thought that he'd never amount to anything. When I asked what the plan was, his core belief about himself led him to hear what he *perceived* to be what I thought of him as opposed to what I actually asked.

Cognitive behavioral therapy can help change one's core beliefs about themselves, so that the negative thought patterns that we develop can begin to dissipate.

## Biofeedback

Biofeedback is essentially monitoring the body and providing information through audio or visual feedback. Anxiety disorders are often accompanied by physical symptoms; recognizing and subsequently altering these through biofeedback may relieve the associated psychological symptoms.[3]

Cody never tried biofeedback, and I can't say that I know anyone who has. (That I know of, anyway.) Nonetheless, it's a common tool for many in their strategy to overcome chronic anxiety. Proponents of biofeedback say it is an excellent tool for overcoming denial and it promotes self-regulation skills, and in a survey study, electroencephalogram neurofeedback—measuring brain waves—was the most common for anxiety. Sixty-five percent of studies found a statistically significant level of symptom reduction. One study of heart rate variability biofeedback, which asked participants to sync pulse and breathing, showed a reduction in self-reported anxiety and a 75 percent drop in stress.[4]

This method may be worth a try if you've already tried other therapies and are looking for something new.

## Exposure Therapy

Feeling anxious isn't a pleasant sensation, so it's totally normal for teens who experience chronic anxiety to want to avoid it if they can. One of the ways they do this is by steering clear of situations they know would elevate their anxiety and purposely go out of their way to avoid doing things they're uncomfortable with.

For example, if your teen has a fear of heights, you might drive out of your way to avoid crossing a tall bridge if they're in the car. Or if the prospect of public speaking leaves them feeling physically ill, they might skip their communications class to avoid doing that project.

Aside from the extreme inconvenience factor, the problem with avoiding fears is that your teen doesn't give themselves the chance to overcome them. The pattern of avoidance strengthens the anxiety response and reinforces it—exposure therapy literally exposes the participant to the situations or objects they're afraid of. Small to large gains with exposure helps to realistically reinforce positive behaviors realistically, and through repeated exposure, they'll (hopefully) feel an increasing sense of control over the situations they dread, and their anxiety will slowly diminish.

Your teen can work on exposure therapy (if it applies) in one of two ways: their therapist may ask them to close their eyes and imagine the scary situation, or they may purposely choose to confront such a situation in real life.

There were many things that Cody wouldn't do during the height of his anxiety. Fear of heights was something he'd always had, and it was extreme: we couldn't go for a drive up a mountain without succumbing to tears. (He can do this now.) He also avoided things like driving and applying for jobs, because driving was scary and applying for jobs meant speaking to adults he didn't know and asking them for something. As time went on, and his medication was regulated, he was able to force himself to do these things, and as a result, they became easier.

Another example of the exposure therapy theory is one involving myself. I had a pretty big fear of spiders until I was in my midtwenties. You know what helped me get over it? Having to hold spiders or capture them from the house and put them outside so Cody would see it would be okay when he was little. My desire to not pass along that fear to my child led to repeated exposure which, in turn, led to the fear going away.

Motivation goes a long way when it comes to exposure therapy. Here are some ways to help your teen get started:

- Reward brave behavior.
- Recognize when they move in the right direction, even if it's small.
- Show by example: expose yourself to something you fear, and ask them to follow your lead.

## Exercise and Yoga

"Available reviews of a wide range of yoga practices suggest they can reduce the impact of exaggerated stress responses and may be helpful for both anxiety and depression."[5]

### Exercise

We often forget how valuable exercise is for our brains, not just our bodies. Sure, exercise helps to maintain a healthy body weight, build muscle, and train the heart and lungs. It lowers blood pressure and even helps prevent diabetes, heart disease, and certain cancers. But it also helps release endorphins (natural painkillers), improves sleep quality, and boosts mood.

A 2013 study found a contrary relationship between anxiety sensitivity and exercise frequency. Researchers suggested that this relationship was due to "avoidance of the physiological sensations of exercise that may be interpreted as anxiety and panic."[6]

In layman's terms, this means that lack of exercise is strongly correlated with increased anxiety.

### Yoga

By reducing perceived stress and anxiety, yoga has been proven to modulate stress response systems in the brain. This, in turn, decreases physiological arousal, such as reducing the heart rate, lowering blood pressure, and easing respiration. There is also convincing evidence that keeping a consistent yoga practice helps to increase heart rate variability, an indicator of the body's ability to respond to stress more compliantly.[7]

Exploring ways your teen can become more physically active could greatly assist them in eradicating at least some of their anxiety symptoms. Again, cardiovascular exercise can help relieve frustration and stress, while yoga trains the brain to relax, promotes self-love, and emphasizes deep breathing (which increases oxygen to the brain).

Which brings us to . . .

## Meditation and the Breath

"Mindfulness training, which includes elements of meditation, body scanning, mindful breathing, and developing a less attached attitude toward one's thoughts, was found to be effective both generally and in three subgroups, including minority children, inner-city youths, and teens with social anxiety."[8]

We touched on this earlier in the book, but in my own opinion, it's worthy of a comeback.

The word *mindfulness* has become somewhat trendy of late, no doubt in response to the current, global need to more accurately understand mental health and its role in current societal issues. Essentially, it's the increasingly popular practice of focusing awareness on the moment by allowing ourselves to be present for consistent, short periods of time—and this is where meditation becomes a factor.

Meditation is essentially the act of being mindful and in the moment.

For some teenagers, the simple act of sitting still for even five minutes can seem incredibly daunting. The world is always busy, and today's teens have grown up in a very fast-paced, global environment where being still translates to feelings of exclusion. There's even a term for it: fear of missing out—the popularly used acronym is FOMO.

But small amounts of consistent meditation have been hailed by successful business leaders (such as Richard Branson and Oprah)[9] and physicians, alike. The benefits of consciously quieting one's mind for only five minutes even just once or twice a day are becoming more and more apparent.

When I asked Cody about meditation, he surprised me by revealing he'd started doing it on his own a while ago. He explained that, in simple terms, it made him feel happier.

Here are some benefits your teen may receive from adding meditation to his daily routine:

- Increased oxygen to the brain
- Better memory, empathy, and decision-making
- Increased positive sense of self
- Increased emotion management
- Increased awareness
- Decreased stress
- Better brain connectivity
- Increased relaxation

## Labyrinth Therapy

I've recently become educated on the concept of "labyrinth therapy." Essentially, the process involves walking a labyrinth for the purpose of mindfulness.

Not to be confused with a maze, a labyrinth represents the intertwined nature of the journey and the goal in healing—the means incorporates the end; the walk is the meditation. Therefore, labyrinth therapy involves both journey and goal.

Walking a labyrinth can be very therapeutic if the meaning behind it can be received by the participant. This technique in intentional stress relief goes back thousands of years and seems to be making a comeback of late. Some cities have labyrinths installed into parks for this purpose, but if yours doesn't, you can simply create one by mowing a pattern into your grass at home or using rocks and stones to make an outline.

This could be a fun and fulfilling project for the whole family to participate in or could be something special that your teenager wants to create for themselves or others.

## Aromatherapy

There is a definite connection between scent and emotion due to neuroanatomy. The part of the brain associated with smell is in close proximity to the part of the brain associated with memory. Some smells trigger memories that are pleasant (or not), and others we deem to be simply enjoyable (or not). Scent is so important to us, that there's even a connection between losing one's olfactory sense and depression.[10]

Knowing this, why not use scents to our advantage when it comes to improving our feelings of anxiety?

There are many natural scents that are known to curb anxiousness, like bergamot, lemon, and lavender. In fact, a 2010 multicenter, double-blind, randomized study found that lavender oil is as effective as lorazepam (a benzodiazepine medication commonly used to treat anxiety) in people with generalized anxiety disorder.[11]

Errr . . . *that's* kind of amazing.

Cody has always been drawn to certain smells and strongly put off by others. When I became more educated on the positive effects that aromatherapy (basically, using certain essential oils to frame the scent of one's environment) has on mood, so did he—and it's interesting to find out what people will choose when it comes to smells they enjoy.

Cody chose scents that were naturally antianxiety without even realizing it; oils like lemon, orange, and peppermint were his go-to smells when we made rollers together. We would use rollers to spread essential oil on our necks and wrists and inhale the scents that made us feel good. We'd also dilute the oils in water and diffuse them in the spaces we hung out in.

Here are some essential oils that are known to help lessen anxiety when diffused:[12]

- Bergamot
- Chamomile
- Lavender
- Lemon
- Lemon balm
- Orange
- Rose
- Rosemary
- Yarrow

Later on, we'll further discuss the role of medicinal herbs like the ones listed.

## Nutritional Therapy

"Nutritional and herbal supplementation is an effective method for treating anxiety and anxiety-related conditions without the risk of serious side effects."[13]

You've probably heard the phrase "you are what you eat," right? While it may not be exactly true (none of us resembles a hamburger or a head of lettuce), our physical, mental, and spiritual health is all very much affected by the foods we choose to fuel our bodies with. Every single day, we make a choice to eat for good health or not—it's that simple.

What's *not* simple is trying to make good choices when your mental health is already heavily affected by anxiety. We've already touched on the fact that teens who suffer from chronic anxiety often can't eat at regular times of the day or sometimes at all, due to other physical manifestations of their disorder. It's so important to make food count: every little bit can either help or hinder one's mood.

Here are some tips on how to help your teen utilize food to aid in recovery from anxiety:

Do

- Eat at regular times throughout the day.
- Consume several small meals over a few large ones.
- Elect leafy greens, fibrous fruits and veggies, and plant-based proteins.
- Choose whole grains over processed ones.
- Reduce sugar intake.
- Limit alcohol and caffeine.
- Incorporate specific supplements (coming up next!).

Don't

- Wait until hunger is overwhelming to eat.
- Skip meals.
- Eat just before bed.
- Binge on empty calories (foods that have no nutritional value, such as sugary cereals).

- Consume foods that are known to induce "brain fog." (Wondering what brain fog is? Basically, it's a broad term for dysfunctions in focus, learning, and memory that can induce brief episodes of confusion, disorientation, frustration, and, ultimately, anxiety.)

## Supplements

The results from a study on the benefits of nutritional and herbal supplements for anxiety and anxiety-related disorders state the following:

"Natural remedies have been used for centuries in many cultures to alleviate anxiety and its symptoms with surprising effectiveness. In Western cultures, however, research that proves the usefulness of medicinal herbs and natural substances has only begun to gain momentum over the past few decades. In addition, the absence of proper guidelines governing the production and use of vitamins, minerals, amino acids, and herbs for medicinal purposes is also causing the clinical prescription of these natural treatments to lag behind in the United States."[14]

Although dietary supplements are never a replacement for actual food, they can assist your teenager in obtaining the nutrients they require while they work on lowering their anxiety levels and getting their diet back on track. Your doctor can also help you identify or confirm any deficiencies (typically via blood testing), as well as offer information on dosage and overall dietary health.

Several common supplements help to alleviate symptoms of anxiety:

### Vitamin A

People with anxiety sometimes lack this vitamin. Vitamin A is an antioxidant that's been shown to help manage anxiety symptoms.

### B-complex

B-complex supplements contain all the B vitamins that your body needs, and many are essential to a healthy nervous system. Increasing vitamin B12 can help improve symptoms of anxiety and depression.[15]

## Vitamin C

Antioxidants like vitamin C can help prevent oxidative damage (which can cause anxiety) in your nervous system.[16]

## Vitamin D

Vitamin D is an important nutrient that helps the body absorb other vitamins. Vitamin D deficiency can lead to other vitamin deficiencies, which may compound anxiety and make it worse. People who live in the north are more susceptible to a vitamin D deficiency than those who reside in sunny areas of the world.

## Vitamin E

Vitamin E is another antioxidant. Your body uses this nutrient up quickly in times of stress and anxiety, so for those who are chronically anxious, taking this supplement regularly is a good idea. Supplemental vitamin E may help restore this balance and reduce your symptoms.

## Omega Fatty Acids

Fish oil, walnuts, and ground flax seed* are high in omega-3 fatty acids, which are antioxidants. Omega-3 supplements like EPA and DHA have been shown to help reduce anxiety.

*Note that ground flax can help regulate bowel movements if constipation is an issue, so if it is, you'd be helping your teen kill two birds with one stone (so to speak).

## Magnesium

Magnesium is a necessary mineral for human health, and your body doesn't need very much of it. However, if you aren't getting enough, magnesium deficiency may lead to symptoms of anxiety, such as sleep disturbances.

Keep in mind that this is not a comprehensive list; ask your doctor about other types of supplements that may be useful in assisting your teen in recovery from anxiety.

## Floatation Therapy

If you haven't yet heard of floatation therapy, you're in for a treat. It is what it sounds like: you float (in body-temperature water, in the dark, with neutral scents and no sound for usually about ninety minutes).

The idea is that by depriving your entire body of external stimuli, it gives you the opportunity to relax and turn your brain off. Specifically, the practice helps treat anxiety by encouraging changes in the body and mind. It works to offer deep relaxation and physical changes to help people feel refreshed and revitalized.

Here are three ways that floating may help your teen to relax and induce calm thoughts:

### Lowering Cortisol

Cortisol is known as the stress hormone. It's a natural chemical the body produces in times of stress like after car accidents or during a fight. However, our busy modern lives also cause higher cortisol levels. Stress from relationships, work, and even travel can cause serious effects. Floatation has been linked to huge reductions in the amount of cortisol in your body, which reduces anxiety and can also assist in other ways that high cortisol may be affecting you.

### Lower Blood Pressure

Stress has a lasting impact on blood pressure, as well. Elevated blood pressure can cause heart damage and may lead to eventual heart disease. Floatation encourages blood vessels to dilate, reducing the pressure and allowing the heart to work more easily. This helps prevent long-term issues and also builds a greater sense of wellness, which in turn, further reduces stress.

### Catharsis of Stressful Thoughts

Many of our stressful thoughts are induced by our loud and busy environments. Staring at screens and working long hours can keep your mind wound up with no means to come back down.

In a floatation tank, there's no external stimulation. There's no sense of temperature, sound, scent, or light. No ringing phones or bill payments can reach you. When you're floating, you can let go of everything else and focus on allowing your mind to unwind, bringing a deep sense of relaxation.

## Singing and Music Therapy

*Time* magazine published an article in 2013 called "Singing Changes Your Brain."[17] The author of the work wrote, "Researchers are beginning to discover that singing is like an infusion of the perfect tranquilizer, the kind that both soothes your nerves and elevates your spirits. The elation may come from endorphins, a hormone released by singing, which is associated with feelings of pleasure. Or it might be from oxytocin, another hormone released during singing, which has been found to alleviate anxiety and stress."[18]

It may sound silly, but if your teen enjoys singing, the activity may be one you can promote to them as much as possible. Perhaps singing lessons or joining the school choir or participating in the local community church choir?

Similarly, just listening to music can be incredibly stress and anxiety reducing. The effects of music have been documented by scientists for years, and despite its mysteriousness, we know without a doubt that listening to music activates our entire brains, creating the potential for us to use music to improve the way we think, behave, and feel.

This is where music therapy comes in.

According to the American Music Therapy Association, music therapy can have profound effects and has helped many people since it became an established profession in the 1950s.

Music therapists work with individuals of all ages to help them communicate more effectively, process difficult experiences, and improve motor or cognitive functioning. A music therapy session is an interactive music-making experience where the client is given musical instruments (including their voice) to use in either an exploratory manner or through a more personalized exercise designed by the therapist to address a specific issue.

If music therapy doesn't sound like something you'll be able to convince your teen to try, you can always suggest they create their own music playlist to use as a tool when attempting to redirect themselves when they begin to feel anxious. By mindfully creating a selection of music, your teen can use a playlist to combat stress, achieve relaxation, increase motivation, and evoke positive emotions.

Here are some guidelines for someone interested in creating a therapeutic playlist:

## Choose Music You Already Love

Start with your own music collection. Your previous associations with pieces of music determine how you'll respond to them. Memories (especially emotional memories) are stimulated by music and can take us back in time in a split second. You've already labeled certain music as happy, sad, energizing, disturbing, and so on. Trust yourself and how you believe songs will make you feel.

Once you identify what it is about music that makes you feel a certain way, you may want to supplement your current collection by finding new music that contains similar characteristics. Place pieces of music into different categories according to your common moods.

## Listen to What You Enjoy

Only listen to music you love. You know what you like and should be able to find enough variety within your preferred music to match different moods. (You wouldn't be choosing the same music as your teen, and they wouldn't choose yours. This is a very personal playlist!)

## Find Music That Evokes Inspiration

As humans, we are constantly striving to be understood. This could explain why we tend to enjoy music that we find relatable or music that speaks to us in one way or another. Songs can validate our feelings and provide comfort when they match our mood.

For instance, listening to sad music actually causes our brains to produce the same neurochemical that is released when we cry. This chemical (prolactin) helps to elicit feelings of comfort, meaning that listening to a sad song when we are feeling down not only provides empathy, it also causes our brain to try to make us feel better.

## Match Your Mood

Consider how you feel right now. Is your heart racing, or are you feeling slow? Are you feeling heavy? How fast are you breathing? Before trying to change your mood with music, you'll need to match it. This is easier done when you can consider different musical elements:

**Tempo:** Pick a piece of music that matches your heartbeat, your breathing, and how fast you feel you are moving.

**Volume:** Are you feeling loud or soft? If you are overstimulated and feel like you need to turn everything off, first find the music that matches your current state. Find a song with soft lyrics and instruments.

Perhaps you are lacking energy and motivation and things around you are quiet. Search for a song with an upbeat tempo that invigorates you!

**Harmony:** Musical instrumentation and background vocals are often written to blend nicely with a melody to add layers of sound in a tonal structure. Some music actually uses instruments and tight harmonies that create a feeling of tension or conflict. Think about your perceived level of stress and how tense you might feel.

Also, think about the instruments that appeal to you in the moment.

## Try Music Without Lyrics

Song lyrics leave a little less up to the imagination because someone else's story is being told. When lyrics are included in a piece of music, more of our brains are used to process these lyrics. If you're using music for the purpose of trying to relax, you may want to allow your mind to wander without consciously focusing on the music. This is more challenging when lyrics are involved. So try no lyrics!

## Create Lists that Match Your Intended Mood

Consider your goal: do you want to feel energetic, happy, relaxed, or optimistic after listening to your playlist? With your intended mood in mind, think of how you might organize songs to bring you from your current emotional state to your desired one. For example, if you started with an up-tempo piece of music that matched your initial state of heightened anxiety, find something a little slower for your next song. If you are trying to move toward a more relaxed state, select a piece of music that is slightly slower for your third song. The third piece should also have less instrumentation or fewer vocals.

The goal is to decrease the amount of stimulation in the music so your playlist can facilitate a gradual transition from a state of anxious to calm while allowing you time to adjust to the music. Select songs that are two to four minutes long, and make sure your playlist contains at least half an hour of music. You want to give your body plenty of time to experience your current emotion and adjust physiologically with the music.

### Trust Your Musical Intuition

If you've ever listened to music and began to cry or were motivated to run an extra few minutes because of it, then you know that music can have an extreme impact on emotions. When intended, music can provide comfort during difficult times and also promote relaxation. Although there is much to consider when using music therapeutically, humans have a particular knack for choosing music that soothes and heals them, without having to think too much about the technical aspects.

Trust yourself, and if you feel you might need more assistance with this process, consider consulting with a board-certified music therapist.

## Ingesting Medicinal Herbs

Aside from supplements, there are many medicinal herbs that, in the correct recommended dosage, can help increase levels of certain vitamins and minerals and help to ease symptoms of anxiety. These herbs include the following:

### Valerian Root

Valerian root encourages relaxation and is commonly used as a sleep aid for insomnia (which, as you now know, is a pretty common by-product of anxiety). Aside from helping one sleep, the root is a natural remedy for anxiety.

### Kava

A well-known antianxiety remedy, kava (or kava root) promotes relaxation. It's most frequently consumed in pill form, though it can also be found in liquid. Some key benefits from the consumption of kava root are muscle relaxation and improved cognitive function.

The use of kava as a treatment for generalized anxiety has been reviewed in several studies and found to be an effective and safe treatment.[19] (The natural supplement has been reported to interact with alcohol negatively, but if your teen is trying to lessen his anxiety, it's probably best that alcohol be avoided, anyway.)

## Ashwagandha

This adaptogenic herb has traditionally been used to treat anxiety and diluted energy. Ashwagandha helps to balance the hormones that contribute to anxiety as well as help induce relaxation and aid sleep.[20] It's ingested most commonly in pill form or consumed as a tea.

Cody raves about the antianxiety benefits of taking this herb once a day in pill form.

## Rhodiola

Like ashwagandha, rhodiola can have a positive effect on your teen's stress levels and their ability to control and manage stress. This herb has been shown to have beneficial qualities in the relief of anxiety symptoms and encourages calmness and relaxation.[21]

## Passionflower

This beautiful flower is used as a natural medicine for anxiety sufferers. Passionflower has a calming effect on those feeling restless and anxious.

In a study titled "Nutritional and Herbal Supplements for Anxiety and Anxiety-Related Disorders," researchers concluded that "passionflower is as effective as benzodiazepines in eliminating anxiety symptoms."[22]

Note: It's known to cause drowsiness, so it's best to take this herb before going to bed.

## Chamomile

Sipping a cup of chamomile tea before bed to induce relaxation is probably something you've either already done or at least heard of. Chamomile is a gentle, effective, and natural way to treat anxiety. It's also been known to ease digestion issues and encourage sleep, assisting those who might suffer from anxiety-induced insomnia.

## Lemon Balm

Lemon balm is lovely to smell—in the past, Cody and I have grown it in our backyard garden and used to pluck leaves to rub between our fingers and inhale deeply to benefit from its fresh, clean scent.

As a natural anxiety remedy, it's been used for thousands of years to help relieve anxiety symptoms and encourage relaxation. Lemon balm may also be helpful in treating gastrointestinal issues and headaches. Several studies have found that lemon balm, known for its calming and soothing properties, not only helps in relieving anxiety but can also improve mood and reduce stress.

## Animal Therapy

An emotional support animal is one that eases the emotional or psychological symptoms associated with the owner's condition or disorder. Just by being present and sensing their human's moods, these animals can help pacify their caregiver's emotional upsets. They act as a constant friend and companion to their owners and help them cope with their emotional issues, which can help their owners cope with everyday matters.

Animals (traditionally horses, dogs, and cats) can provide support for emotional and mood disorders, including anxiety, depression, post-traumatic stress disorder, and more by simply being present when their owner becomes emotionally distraught.[23]

It wasn't the original intention, but in the spring of 2017, our family took home a golden retriever that we named Grover. Cody didn't come for the drive to pick him up because it was two hours each way, and he couldn't handle being isolated in the car for that long. (He still hates to be in the car for long periods of time.) When we arrived home, we announced the new puppy's name to Cody, who frowned in obvious disagreement, and immediately stated he'd call him Mister Peanut Butter instead—a name that totally stuck.

Although the pup was meant to distract and provide some emotional comfort for my younger two children (whose father and I were about to separate), he ended up mostly providing emotional support for Cody and his escalating anxiety. Over the first two years, this dog received more hugs from my older son than he did from anyone else—and believe me, this dog was loved *hard*. Cody and Mister Peanut Butter slept together, went for walks together several times each day, and played endlessly. This beautiful canine always knew (still knows) when Cody was down, and Cody reaped the benefits of having such an emotionally attentive animal in his life.

I asked Cody while we were writing this book if he felt the dog had been like a therapy animal for him, and he immediately replied yes. There's just something about pets, and research can confirm this.

In fact, a 2016 study concluded that "pets should be considered a main rather than a marginal source of support in the management of long-term mental health problems."[24]

Aside from dogs, other animals have been proven therapeutic for people suffering from mental health disorders such as anxiety. Horses, cats, rabbits, and even birds can help people settle down and focus on something other than themselves. And taking care of another living being can be powerful and extremely gratifying.

## Chapter Summary

Here's a summary of some of the ways you can encourage your teen to cope with anxiety, naturally:

- Discuss cognitive behavioral therapy (CBT).
- Attempt exposure therapy, if applicable.
- Increase your teen's cardiovascular exercise.
- Introduce yoga, meditation, and conscious breathing.
- Find or create a labyrinth.
- Explore aromatherapy.
- Try encouraging your teen to sing more.
- Make a playlist that can help lessen your teen's anxiety.
- Introduce floatation therapy.
- Provide your teen with healthy food, and be consistent.
- Include appropriate supplements and medicinal herbs.
- Consider animal therapy.

# 10

# MEDICATION FOR ANXIETY

> "Approximately 8% of teens ages thirteen to eighteen years have [been diagnosed with] an anxiety disorder, with symptoms commonly emerging around age six. Unfortunately, only about 18% of these youth receive the mental health care they need."[1]

THIS chapter may be somewhat controversial. Like I once was, you may feel strongly that your teen should not be introduced to commercial pharmaceuticals to aid his anxiety. I totally understand that—I was there, myself. Whether or not to explore medication is a very personal decision and should be fully discussed with your teen and your family doctor.

That aside, I have to admit that the medication my son is currently taking while we're writing this book (and has been taking for months now) has been a complete game changer for him and our entire family. I won't try to talk you into the medication route because I can't tell you that mood-altering medication is for your child—it may not be, and many experts champion the act of avoiding it.

But it may be an option for your teen, so I'm going to go ahead with this chapter.

Medications prescribed for anxiety and stress disorders fall into several different categories. The most commonly prescribed medications are antidepressants (since anxiety and depression often hold hands, this makes sense) and benzodiazepines.

It's important to note that good physicians treat teenagers very carefully when it comes to prescribing these types of medications. Although treatment and resolution of a disorder like chronic anxiety is incredibly important, there have been many studies that examine what effects drugs like selective serotonin reuptake inhibitors (SSRIs) have on the still-developing teenage brain. Because of this, many doctors will err on the side of caution when developing a treatment plan for teens, and although meds are a possibility, natural treatments like cognitive behavioral therapy, a consistent movement regime (yoga and another exercise), and a strong suggestion to refrain from recreational drugs and over-the-counter medications are typically explored first.

When someone is suffering from severe depression, the lack of energy is often what keeps that individual from acting upon suicidal thoughts, also known as suicidal ideation. As one is treated for their disorder, that person typically gains energy, and the volition to commit suicide can increase along with that energy. Suddenly there's an individual who generally feels better and has more energy, but when those suicidal thoughts do come—even if they're being produced much less frequently than before treatment—the person has the stamina to act on them. With teens, this is a major concern because of their incomplete brain development.

An adult with a fully formed brain might recognize the process or may have been coached on what to expect and told they only need to hang on and get past this stage. But a teen doesn't think in the same logical way—their developing brains are emotional and still largely unregulated—and this can be a scary situation: *elevated energy does not equal reduced suicidal ideation*.

Conclusions following a recent study in which researchers assessed adults' and teens' aggression and suicidal tendencies confirmed that "in adults there was no significant increase . . . but in children and adolescents the risk of suicidality and aggression doubled."[2]

*This* is what deters many physicians from prescribing mood-altering medications to teenagers.

That all being said, the SSRIs that Cody is currently taking while I'm writing these words have been an incredible gift—a literal lifesaver. Within the first six weeks, this is what happened:

- His energy increased.
- His sleep schedule became much more regular.
- His appetite came back.
- He gained some weight.

And this is what has transpired in the months that followed:

- He became goofy and funny again.
- He hangs out with the family more.
- He's overall more pleasant to be around.
- He's more helpful at home.
- He's showing interest in getting a job and actually applied for a few.
- He's put himself in a few uncomfortable situations that he wouldn't have before.
- He's hanging around with better friends.
- His self-awareness has increased—*a lot.*

## Cody's Experience with Antianxiety Medication

I always thought commercial meds for anxiety were stupid until one worked. But I needed to take it with low expectations, and it didn't work alone. Eating better, working out, and abstaining from drugs was important. All of these factors together contributed to finally experiencing success in an antianxiety medication leveling my mood.

I found that I needed to let go of the control I wanted to have in the process and the actual medication itself. I refused meds for a long time because I was focused on trying to get what I wanted, which were uppers or stimulants. I thought being prescribed

Adderall was my ticket to feeling better, and I was so angry when doctors wouldn't give me a prescription for that.

Now I understand.

Adderall would have been a temporary solution to what needed to be more permanent. Yes, I wanted energy and to feel high and happy, but I needed to have my brain chemistry sorted out.

For those who have never been on medication for mood disorders, there are side effects. The first time I was ever prescribed an SNRI, I lasted two weeks and then took myself off cold turkey because I didn't like how they made me feel.

That wasn't a good idea.

It was more than a year later that I finally began taking an SSRI that would eventually help level me out a lot. There were side effects to this medication too, but I was better prepared for them and in a place where I knew I needed help. Side effects included feeling a bit high or drowsy at different times of the day or more awake at certain times. It messed up my wake/sleep schedule at first, and I found myself really tired in the afternoons and awake throughout the night. I also felt kind of sick or not hungry.

It took about a month to get used to the medication, and then every time we increased my dosage by five milligrams, it took a couple of weeks to adjust.

You also have to be pretty self-aware and recognize when it's the right or wrong time for a dosage increase. My family doctor started me on five milligrams of an antidepressant. After about six weeks, I began to take ten milligrams. Two months after that, my dosage was increased to fifteen, but after a few days, I realized I wasn't ready for the increase and brought myself back down to ten. Eventually, I increased to fifteen when I felt I was ready, and it worked better.

So you have to pay attention.

Overall, I can honestly say that this medication has made a massive difference for me. I sleep better, I've gained weight, and I feel motivated. My relationship with my family got better, and I feel like myself again.

I think for teens who need mood-altering meds, the key is to understand the way they work, expect the side effects and know they're temporary, and to agree to cut out other substances that are being used to alter mood. That last one's hard because if you know you can feel better right away by taking something, why wouldn't you?

But it's temporary—and the long-term advantage of quitting drugs and sticking to a program that's recommended by a doctor is what will actually help. Teenagers have a tough time looking into the future, but that's what you have to do if you want to feel better.

## Common Medications for Anxiety

There are five main classes of drugs that doctors prescribe to treat depression and anxiety. All of them work in different ways with the neurotransmitters your teenager already has in his brain—so let's get biological.

It's a common misconception that medications prescribed for anxiety and/or depression supply extra serotonin or dopamine. In fact, the medication simply allows our brain to function differently to use the chemicals we already possess better.

Receptors in the brain responsible for regulating chemicals like serotonin and dopamine may let too much of the chemical pass through to the bloodstream. By employing the help of an inhibitor (more explanation follows), these receptors become regulated and subsequently begin to streamline the proper amount of what is already accessible.

The following medications are listed in order of most popular to least when prescribed for anxiety:

### Selective Serotonin Reuptake Inhibitors (SSRIs)

SSRIs ease depression by adjusting available levels of serotonin in the brain. Serotonin is one of the chemical messengers (neurotransmitters) that carry signals between brain cells, and the SSRIs block the reuptake of serotonin in the brain, making more serotonin available and using the chemicals more productively.

SSRIs are termed "selective" because they seem primarily to affect serotonin, not other neurotransmitters. They're commonly used to treat both depression and anxiety disorders.

All SSRIs work in a similar way and generally can cause similar side effects, though some people may not experience any. Many side effects may go away after the first few weeks of treatment; others may lead you and your doctor to try a different drug. If your teen can't tolerate one SSRI, they may be able to tolerate a different one, as SSRIs differ in chemical makeup.

Possible side effects of SSRIs may include the following:

- Drowsiness
- Nausea
- Dry mouth
- Insomnia
- Diarrhea
- Nervousness, agitation, or restlessness
- Dizziness
- Erectile dysfunction
- Headache[3]
- Blurred vision

## Serotonin-Norepinephrine Reuptake Inhibitors (SNRIs)

SNRIs are a class of medications that are also effective in treating depression. They're also sometimes used to treat other conditions, such as anxiety disorders and long-term (chronic) pain. For this reason, SNRIs may be helpful if you have chronic pain in addition to depression or anxiety.

SNRIs can help ease anxiety by impacting chemical messengers (neurotransmitters) used to communicate between brain cells. They work by ultimately effecting changes in brain chemistry and communication in brain nerve cell circuitry known to regulate mood and block the reabsorption of serotonin and norepinephrine in the brain.

All SNRIs work in a similar way and generally can cause similar side effects, though some people may not experience any side effects. Side effects are usually mild and go away after the first few weeks of treatment. If prescribed an SNRI, your teen may be advised to take the medication with food to prevent or reduce nausea. If your teen can't tolerate one SNRI, they may be able to tolerate a different one, as each SNRI varies in chemical makeup.

The most common possible side effects of SNRIs include the following:

- Nausea
- Dry mouth
- Dizziness
- Headache
- Excessive sweating

Other possible side effects may include the following:

- Tiredness
- Constipation
- Insomnia
- Changes in sexual function
- Loss of appetite[4]

## Noradrenergic and Specific Serotonergic Antidepressant (NaSSA)

NaSSAs block negative feedback effects on norepinephrine and serotonin secretion by the presynaptic cell. This action increases the concentrations of these neurotransmitters in the synaptic cleft to bring them to a normal range. They also block some serotonin receptors on the postsynaptic cell, which enhances serotonin neurotransmission.[5]

The most common side effects include the following:

- Drowsiness
- Dry mouth
- Increased appetite
- Weight gain

It's extremely important to understand that reducing or stopping usage of any dosage of any mood-altering medication must be coordinated under the guidance of a medical professional. There can be dire consequences for taking oneself off medications like the ones listed above without a professional plan in place.

## Questioning Big Pharma

Pharmacological companies do not have a good rap, and most parents I've spoken with about their feelings concerning antianxiety medications for youths seem to be very aware of this. Major pharmaceutical companies are rather infamous for being known to bury bad news, which has had an effect on people's health, and therefore their lives. Whether it's not testing new drugs properly (as with the case of thalidomide, which was discovered to cause birth defects) or restricting publication of results indicating that Paxil caused an increase in suicide risk for teens,[6] Big Pharma has taken some hits in regards to the trust of the general public.

But that doesn't mean antianxiety medication should be ruled out: untreated chronic anxiety disorders put teens at risk of lower school performance, poor social skills, and risky behaviors like substance abuse.[7]

When considering anxiety medication for your teenager, write down a list of questions you have and bring them to your teen's doctor or mental health professional. Some of these might include the following:

- How long will the medication take to be fully effective?
- What side effects are most common?
- Will the side effects subside after a period of time?
- Are there any health risks associated with taking this medication?
- Are there any negative side effects commonly associated with discontinuing the medication?
- Will this medication interact negatively with any other medications my teen is taking?
- Are there any lifestyle changes that need to be made before commencing pharmaceutical intervention?

It may take several attempts to find the right medication for your teen, and these needs may change over time. Some medications can take up to a month to achieve their full effect and for a doctor and your teenager to determine whether they are working effectively.

## Chapter Summary

Here's what you can do to begin the conversation with your teen about possible medical intervention, should you feel it's an appropriate topic to explore:

- Loop in your family doctor or counselor.
- Ask your teen what they think about the idea.
- Research medications with your teen.
- Find a good doctor to discuss this option with (one who discusses it at length with you and your teen and doesn't just haphazardly throw around a prescription pad).
- Try and determine whether to go straight to medication or provide your teen with therapy or counseling with a qualified therapist first.

# 11

## SELF-HARM AND SUICIDE

"Suicide is the third-leading cause of death—after accidents and homicide—among teens and young adults between fifteen and twenty-four years of age."[1]

WE touched on the possibility of self-harm in the previous chapter, but this chapter will explain an anxiety-ridden teen's tendency toward it—and suicide—in better detail.

First of all, let's get this straight: self-harm and suicide are completely different. If death occurs as a result of self-harm, it's an accident. Self-harm is to cope and distract; suicide is the intent to end one's life.

The motivations are completely different between the two.

Self-harm is a hard sign of severe emotional distress. Teens engage in this harmful behavior to relieve feelings of stress, anxiety, or emotional pain. Self-harm can relieve tension momentarily, which gives teens the false belief that this harmful and unsustainable coping strategy actually works. Some might use it to distract themselves, to avoid processing their emotions, or to simply punish themselves. The physical pain they inflict numbs the emotional pain they're experiencing, and they can often feel like this potentially dangerous practice is helpful.

In reality, the practice is a temporary escape that can result in a lifetime of ineffective coping if they don't learn how to manage their emotional pain in healthier ways. Although teens who engage in this destructive behavior often describe a temporary feeling of relief or even elation, it can also result in an overwhelming feeling of shame and terrible scars that last a lifetime—a visual reminder of emotional and physical pain.

It's not uncommon for teens to be engaging in self-harm long before you know about it, and that's not your fault. But it's important to address it swiftly and seriously once discovered and/or conversed about.

## Common Ways Adolescents Inflict Self-Harm

A study titled "Self-Injurious Behaviors in a College Population"[2] examined the self-injurious behavior of over 2,800 college students. The results? Seventeen percent of the respondents reported self-injurious behavior.

Youths use a variety of ways to inflict hurt upon themselves, but according to the study referred to above, these are the most common ways in which they may attempt to relieve or distract themselves through self-harm:

**Scratching or pinching:** This behavior includes severely scratching or pinching with fingernails or objects to the point that bleeding occurs or marks remain on the skin. This method of self-injury was seen in more than half of all students who reported participating in self-harm.

**Impact with objects:** This self-harm behavior includes banging or punching objects to the point of bruising or bleeding. This way to injure oneself was seen in just over 37 percent of the study's self-harming students.

**Self-impact:** This injury method includes banging or punching oneself to the point of bruising or bleeding. This way to self-injure was seen in almost 25 percent of the students who reported self-harming behaviors.

**Cutting:** Cutting is often considered synonymous with self-harm; this way of self-mutilation occurred in just over one in three students who reported self-harming. Also, cutting was more common among females. While the actual cutting of one's skin can be relieving to those engaged in it, it's also often the sight of the blood itself that can provide a calming visual. (Some therapists allow their patients to draw on their skin with a marker to experience something similar.)

**Ripped skin:** This way to self-mutilate includes ripping or tearing skin and was seen in just under 16 percent of those who admitted to self-harming behaviors.

**Carving:** This is when a person carves words or symbols into the skin. This method of self-mutilation was identified by just under 15 percent of those who intentionally hurt themselves.

**Healing interference:** This way of self-mutilation is often in combination with other types of self-harm. In this case, a person purposefully hampers the healing of wounds. This method of self-harm was used by 13.5 percent of study participants, and examples might be pulling out stitches or picking at scabs.

**Burning of the skin:** Burning skin is a way of self-mutilation and was seen in 12.9 percent of students who self-harmed.

**Rubbing objects into the skin:** This type of self-harm involves the rubbing of sharp objects (such as glass, hard plastic, or small pebbles) into the skin. Twelve percent of responding students used this way to self-harm. People may also embed or insert things like safety pins or staples into the body.

**Hair pulling:** This way to self-harm is medically known as trichotillomania. In trichotillomania, a person feels compelled to pull out their own hair (and/or eyebrows and/or eyelashes) and, in some cases, even ingest that hair. This type of self-injury was seen in 11 percent of students who self-harmed.

**Tattooing and/or piercing:** Tattooing and piercing one's body can also be forms of self-harm. Dassinger conveyed that sometimes she can tell when her patients have had a recent rough patch by noticing new tattoos or piercings. This is also a much more socially acceptable way to self-harm if the tattoos and piercings are being used for that purpose.

**Intentional substance abuse:** Basically, this method of self-harm entails drinking way too much alcohol (probably much too often) and/or smoking, ingesting, or shooting up illicit drugs to blur emotions your teen doesn't want to feel. This form of self-harm can be lethal and is extremely dangerous.

All self-harm methods depend on the motivation behind the behavior and the way your teen chooses to harm themselves doesn't matter as much as why they're doing it in the first place. They may not know that what they're doing can be classified as self-harm. For example, if your teen is biting their nails down to the quick and meticulously pulling out eyebrow hair, they may not realize they're harming themselves as a method of distraction or release.

If you're caring for a chronically anxious teen, chances are good they're harming themselves in one way or another or have thought about it, and this goes back to feeling disconnected while experiencing age-appropriate lack of impulse control and regulation. Signs and symptoms of self-injury are not usually easy to spot, because teens who self-injure become very adept at hiding their scars or explaining them away.

To spot the signs of self-harm, consider if your teenager has

- a preference for wearing concealing clothing at all times, such as long sleeves and pants;
- an avoidance of situations where more revealing clothing might be the norm (like unexplained refusal to go to the beach or a friend's pool party); or
- unusually frequent complaints of accidental injury or clumsiness.

## Self-Harm Statistics

Self-injury statistics show that this disturbing phenomenon is a real and present danger to vulnerable people worldwide, especially in developed countries such as the United States. Frequently untreated depression, anxiety, and other mental health challenges create an environment of despair that leads people to cope with these challenges in unhealthy ways.

Here are some current self-harm statistics taken directly from Healthy Place:[3]

- Each year, one in five females and one in seven males hurt themselves on purpose.
- Nine out of ten people who engage in self-harm begin during their teen or preadolescent years.
- Nearly 50 percent of those who engage in self-injurious activities have been sexually abused.
- Girls encompass 60 percent of those who engage in self-injurious behavior.
- About half of those who engage in self-mutilation begin in their early teens and continue on into adulthood.
- Many of those who self-injure report learning how to from friends or from pro–self-injury websites.
- About two million cases are reported every year in the United States.
- Seventy percent of those who repeatedly self-injure often engage in multiple ways to do so.[4]

## Suicide

> "Nine in ten teens who take their own lives were previously diagnosed with a psychiatric or mental health condition or disorder—more than half of them with a mood disorder such as depression or anxiety."
>
> —American Academy of Pediatrics.[5]

The idea of your own kid deciding that life isn't worth living and acting on that powerful thought definitely falls under the category of "Parents' Worst Nightmares." I remember where I was the very first time Cody said the words "I just want to die." The physical reaction one's body has to a statement like that, coming from your own child, is difficult to explain. Kind of like your lungs being ripped from your chest cavity and at the same time your heart trying to jump out of your throat.

And that's just the physical reaction.

I had no idea that anxiety and suicide were almost as closely related to depression and suicide. Because anxiety and depression are so closely interwoven themselves, I guess this makes sense. But as someone who doesn't experience the level of anxiousness my son did, I didn't know it could be so bad if left untreated or not treated properly.

"Anxiety disorders, especially panic disorder and PTSD, are independently associated with suicide attempts. Clinicians need to assess suicidal behavior among patients presenting with anxiety problems."[6]

The research study referred to above stated within their findings that "among individuals reporting a lifetime history of suicide attempt, over 70 percent had an anxiety disorder. Even after adjusting for sociodemographic factors, the presence of an anxiety disorder was significantly associated with having made a suicide attempt."[7]

So, how can you tell if suicide is something your anxious teenager may be idealizing?

## Warning Signs of an Impending Suicide Attempt

- Being depressed or having other mental disorders
- Talking directly or indirectly about wanting to die or "not be around"
- Increased social isolation and disengaging from commitment
- Significant changes in appearance and hygiene
- Giving away valued possessions; making other preparations for death
- A sudden change in mood

## Risk Factors That Make Suicide More Likely

While the act of successful suicide is always a shocking occurrence for friends and family members to try and process, there are usually (but not always) warning signs that precede such a horrific event. These include the following:

- Previous suicide attempt(s)
- Having a family member or friend who has killed themselves; multiple suicides in the community or peer group
- Other recent, significant losses, such as the loss of a relationship or job
- Cultural and religious beliefs supporting suicide

- Alcohol and drug abuse
- Feelings of hopelessness
- Access to means of suicide (such as a gun or pills)
- Unwillingness to seek help and/or barriers to accessing appropriate mental health treatment

If you feel like a red flag has been raised in regard to a combination of these warning signs and your teen, you need to take it seriously and provide them with immediate professional help.

## Common Misconceptions about Suicide

Because suicide is a very scary premise or idea, it's typically a topic that people tend to avoid or make excuses for. Our brains try to justify the reasoning behind such an act of desperation and/or sadness, and because of this, we often try to remove responsibility and/or make ourselves feel like it's not really an option our kids would choose. We disassociate ourselves from it because the thought of our own teen committing suicide is our absolute worst nightmare.

Here are some misconceptions many of us have about suicide and corresponding information to help educate ourselves on why these statements or ideas aren't true:

- *People who talk about it won't do it.* Wrong—suicide threats should always be taken seriously. The truth is that few individuals are single-minded in their decision to kill themselves; many are asking for help even as they contemplate suicide.
- *People who really want to kill themselves are beyond help.* Not true. Suicidal impulses may be intense but are typically short-lived. The majority of individuals who are suicidal even for extended periods recover and can benefit from treatment.
- *Suicide is a purely personal decision.* This argument is sometimes used to justify a hands-off attitude. It's a misconception because suicide doesn't just affect the person who dies; it affects others also.
- *Asking about suicide can put the idea in someone's mind.* Research proves that this statement is not true.[8] In fact, many people

> having suicidal thoughts often feel relieved when someone asks. Suicidal individuals are engaged in a private struggle with thoughts of death and having someone to talk to that they can trust can make a huge impact. Don't underestimate this.

Talking about the possibility of suicide can alleviate the loneliness of the struggle and can be a first step in obtaining help. Nobody is comfortable with not feeling in control of their own lives, and kids are no different. For teens, feelings of chronic anxiety (and depression) are scary, and they often don't know what's going on or how to get help.

A study that examined the relationship between teens with anxiety, their tendency toward self-medicating, and their subsequent risk for suicide found that "among respondents with an anxiety disorder, self-medication was significantly associated with an increased likelihood of comorbid mood disorders, substance use disorders, distress, suicidal ideation, and suicide attempts. Self-medication behavior remained significantly associated with an increased likelihood of suicidal ideation as well as suicide attempts, even after adjusting for a number of sociodemographic and psychiatric variables. These results suggest that individuals with anxiety disorders who self-medicate their symptoms with alcohol or drugs may be at increased risk for mood and substance use disorders and suicidal behavior."[9]

Let's remember the previous discussion on brain development and anti-anxiety medications.

Recall that an adolescent's brain at around the time of puberty begins to develop very quickly from back to front. This means they make decisions based largely on emotions, not logic—and it's not their fault. It's a biological process that one *cannot* control, which makes the idea of suicide extremely scary, especially when those feelings are coupled with the emergence of a new antianxiety medication.

The Mayo Clinic warns that "in some cases, children, teenagers, and young adults under twenty-five may have an increase in suicidal thoughts or behavior when taking antidepressants."[10] Since antidepressants are commonly prescribed for anxiety, parents of kids who already entertain the idea of self-harm should monitor their teens very carefully if medication is prescribed to them for anxiety, especially within the first few weeks.

Just be aware, parents. My son's medication saved him—saved *us*—but it doesn't work the same for everyone. As long as we're cognizant of the side effects of these meds and can monitor our teens' moods and emotions, we're doing due diligence when it comes to providing care for our kids.

## Tips for Parents on Recognizing and Responding to Self-Harm

As caregivers of anxious teens, what can we do to protect our children from suicidal thoughts and actions? The American Academy of Pediatrics has made the following ten recommendations:[11]

### Don't Do Nothing

As in, don't wait for your teen to get worse to find out if it's real. Assume your observations and gut instincts are correct and begin the conversation. If your teen is showing symptoms of chronic anxiety or depression, action must be taken immediately.

### Pay Attention

Listening to what your teen tells you is important—but it's also important to listen to what they aren't saying.

The American Academy of Pediatrics says that "studies have found that one trait common to families affected by a son's or daughter's suicide is poor communication between parents and child. However, there are usually three or more issues or factors going on all at once in a child's life at the time when he or she is thinking about taking his or her life."[12]

These include the following:

- Breakups
- Family discord or domestic violence
- Family history of suicide
- Impulsiveness and aggressiveness
- Death of a family member or friend
- Chronic pain
- Substance abuse
- Peer pressure

- Access to weapons, such as guns
- Bullying

If you, as a caregiver, note the combination of a few of the above factors, it's a good idea to talk to your child and assess their mental health.

## Take Threats of Suicide Seriously

It's easier to assume that your child is making suicide threats to get a reaction from you rather than wanting actually to die. But here's the thing: Why take the risk? Why assume *anything* when it comes to serious threat of self-harm?

I understand that it's easier said than done. Cody talked about wanting to die a few times, and I was either too shocked and confused to take him seriously, or it happened so often I became desensitized.

Probably both.

But what if he had carried his threats out? After the last time he spoke of taking his own life, I spoke with Dassinger, who advised me simply and firmly to take him to the emergency room the next time he said anything like that, and for two reasons:

1. If he was serious, I would be saving his life.
2. If he wasn't serious, he'd probably stop threatening it if he knew he'd be taken for a mental health assessment each time he did so.

Either way, I was instructed to make the call. Fortunately, Cody hasn't mentioned anything about suicide since, and we haven't had to put ourselves in the proposed situation. But if you encounter this with your teen—they threaten to end their own life—then I suggest doing what Dassinger recommends, taking that threat seriously, and acting on it.

And sometimes it's not a direct suicide comment. Try and be aware of comments that concern you or sound strange (passive suicidal thoughts), such as,

- "Nothing matters."
- "I wonder how many people would come to my funeral?"

- "Sometimes I wish I could just go to sleep and never wake up."
- "Everyone would be better off without me."
- "You won't have to worry about me much longer."[13]

These types of comments, although not direct suicide threats, are definite red flags that should be brought to the attention of a professional. Which brings us to . . .

## Seek Professional Assistance

Here's the deal: as parents and caregivers, it seems like we should know what to do when our kids are struggling, but the fact is, we rarely do, and that's okay. Teens can be intensely private, and that's why we turn to people who do know what to do.

There is zero shame in seeking out a therapist or doctor or crisis center and asking them for help. In fact, there is strength in knowing when something is outside of your realm of expertise and serious enough to warrant a consultation.

## Talk about Your Feelings

Remember: teenagers are still children. They may be taller than you, weigh more than you, and may even have the amazing capability to argue intelligently and make fantastic points during an adult conversation.

But they're still kids, and kids are inexperienced—and this is why it's so important to share yours.

Let your teen know that they aren't alone, that you can relate in some way to what they're going through, and that you'll be here for them, always. Unless you share your own feelings with them, they will assume that they're the only ones to feel what they're currently feeling.

Knowing that others can feel anxious and/or depressed at times gives hope to a situation that for a teen, may seem impossibly difficult.

## Encourage Social Activities

Teenagers learn from interaction with others—from experiences. When anxiety comes into the equation, sometimes the tendency is to lay low to avoid even more discomfort. While it's okay to recognize one's need to turn in every now and again, those with chronic anxiety and/or depression should probably be monitored when it comes to isolating behaviors. If your teen is basically living in their bedroom and only leaving it to use the bathroom or grab the occasional bite to eat, it's up to you to try and draw them out.

As I'm writing this, I'm clearly remembering an example with Cody. It was early afternoon, and he hadn't yet left his bedroom that day. I assumed he was sleeping in, as teens tend to do, but at some point, I knocked on his door and entered to find him curled up in a ball on his bed, sobbing.

He explained that he didn't know what to do and he hadn't been able to leave his room. The anxiety was thick and palpable, and I suggested he come with me to run an errand. I emphasized that all he had to do was brush his teeth and get in the car. Forty-five minutes later, that's what he did.

It took that long to convince him it would be healthy because it would at least get him out and change the course of the afternoon for him. He didn't see any point in coming along with me, because there wasn't one—he just needed to get out of his room to break the cycle of anxiety that was being created in there.

And you know what? It worked.

We ended up running my errand, then going to a shopping center and buying him a few much-needed articles of clothing (this was stressful for him also, and I remember having to bite my tongue and have tons of patience). We stopped at a drive-through and got him something to eat. We were gone for about two hours, and by the time we were home, he was in a good mood. This act of drawing him out and changing the direction of his day and mood was stressful and time-consuming for both of us, but we both knew it had to be done.

Consciously curbing your teenager's tendency to isolate themselves is important, because once they go down that road, it can be difficult to turn back.

## Suggest Exercise

Exercise is incredibly important for everyone, not just teenagers. But teens with anxiety should be especially careful to get in the movement. Exercise (especially cardio) helps to burn feelings of anxiety, rids the body of pent-up energy, increases levels of dopamine, and fosters healthy coping habits.

Here's more information on exercise from the American Academy of Pediatrics:[14]

- Regular exercise causes a gland in the brain to release endorphins (a substance believed to improve mood and ease pain). Endorphins also help by lowering the amount of the stress hormone cortisol in the circulatory system.
- Exercise is an effective distraction for people from their problems and makes us feel better about ourselves.
- Doctors typically recommend working out for at least thirty minutes a day, three or four days a week.
- Any form of exercise that increases the heart rate will do; what matters most is that your teen enjoys the activity and continues to do it on a regular basis.[15]

## Relieve Some Pressure

That is, notice what your teenager is doing and engaged in, and assess whether or not they need to take a few things off their plate. For instance, if your child is engaged in several after-school extracurriculars, perhaps suggest letting a couple of them go.

Or if you know your teen struggles to maintain perfect grades and puts a lot of pressure on themselves, consider talking with them about why they feel pressured and how you can help them get some relief. Maybe let them know they're not expected to do their regular chores during exam week, or maybe add an hour to their curfew.

The idea is simply to provide a little bit of relief.

If *you* are the one putting unnecessary pressure on your child and it's adding to their anxiety, you might need to check yourself. Ask yourself if you're putting pressure on them to perform for them, or for you.

Reassess your own personal need to demand perfection from your child.

## Rid Your Home of Guns

This seems like a no-brainer to me, but I'm Canadian and grew up in Canada—I don't get the gun thing. Americans reading this book may (or may not) have a different experience. Either way, it's important to understand that in a moment of impulsiveness, a suicidal teen could easily make the decision to access a weapon from within the home and carry through an idea made while extremely anxious and/or upset.

Remember that someone who is upset enough to try and kill themselves is not going to care about whether or not they're allowed in the gun case. All it takes is a moment; don't make that moment available—obliterate the opportunity before it even presents itself.

## Have Patience and Show Love

And remind your teen to, too! Mindfully improving one's mental health is hard work and takes dedication and support from the entire household. It won't happen overnight, but it *will* happen. Stick to the plan, supply endless support and love, and both you and your teen will reap the rewards.

### Cody on Anxiety and Self-Harm

I've never felt the urge to hurt myself. I've never cut myself or attempted suicide. The thought of not existing anymore was once appealing to me, but I haven't felt like that in a long time. I know a lot of people who do hurt themselves, and most of them are girls.

Self-harm tactics like cutting is mostly a hidden thing. It's way easier to see pink and angry cuts or thin, white scars of previous, self-inflicted abuse on girls because they're more likely to show their bare legs, stomachs, and full arms.

Anxiety creates an environment of overthinking, so when someone is mean, it fosters anxiety and causes the recipient of the meanness to overthink. Same-sex bullying seems to take place more in grades nine and ten, while opposite-sex bullying takes place more in grades eleven and twelve.

Social media made these situations for teens way worse.

Social media is often used by teens to boost confidence, and then those people get made fun of, which breeds anxiousness. Basically, the harder you try on social media, the shittier your mental health becomes if you're a high schooler.

The worst offender? Instagram—it's a virtual bully ground.

## Chapter Summary

When it comes to self-harm, all methods carry the same message: I'm hurting. It's so important to know what to do if your teen is intentionally harming themselves. Here's a quick summary of that list:

- Understand that self-harm is a giant, red flag.
- Familiarize yourself with the various common methods of ways to hurt oneself.
- Talk to your teen about suicide and know the warning signs.
- If you suspect self-harm of any kind, take action immediately.
- Pay attention to what your teen is saying and also to what they aren't.
- Take threats seriously.
- Seek professional guidance.
- Keep communication lines open.
- Encourage social activities that get your teen talking to others.
- Suggest exercise and show by example.
- Try to relieve some pressure for your teen by being more accommodating than usual.
- Ban guns from your home.
- Have patience and show love.
- Be empathetic and compassionate; don't punish or demean.

**Note:** If you think your teen may be in crisis, you can contact the toll-free National Suicide Prevention Lifeline at 1-800-273-TALK (8255), twenty-four hours a day, seven days a week—the service is available to everyone. The deaf and hard of hearing can contact the lifeline via TTY at 1-800-799-4889. All calls are confidential.

# 12

# CARE FOR THE CAREGIVER

IT took me years to wrap my brain around the fact that the single most important thing you can do for your anxious child is simply be there for them, unconditionally. This sounds easy, right?

It's not.

When you don't understand what anxiety feels like, it can leave you exasperated and impatient. Having to care for a teenager who's experiencing high levels of anxiety is hard. You don't get it, you're mentally exhausted, and it's a long road. You cry a lot.

I cried *a lot*.

Here are some things that people won't tell you about parenting or caring for a teen with chronic anxiety:

- It's terrifying. You're scared for your teen, for your family, and you mourn the loss of what you thought these years might look like.
- You cry a lot. (Okay, I already told you this—but it's true.)
- You feel lost. There is no handbook or manual for how to get

through this, which is why the idea for this book was born. We need to help each other.

- You alienate yourself—but you don't mean to. You live in crisis mode and only put the little energy you have into surviving. You're not thinking about your social status.
- People who haven't gone through it won't understand. Hell, you don't even understand when you're smack in the middle of it! People who bypass this teen situation will not get it—and that's okay. Instead of feeling angry that they don't understand or jealous that they haven't had to go through the experiences related to teen anxiety that you have had to go through, try and be happy for them—dealing with a chronically anxious teen is tough, and you wouldn't wish it on anyone.
- Your own mental health will suffer. You will probably become a little bit depressed. You begin to overthink everything and operate on nerves.
- You don't sleep well. The insomnia that you experience while going through these anxiety years with your teen is unparalleled.

But also . . .

- You learn to appreciate and celebrate little victories. Where once you may have overlooked your teen's smaller accomplishments, you now appreciate *everything.*
- You stop sweating the small stuff. (No milk in the fridge? Who cares?!)
- You become very educated on the topic of anxiety. You begin to read, talk, and immerse yourself in the fascinating (albeit exhausting) land of teenage mental health.
- You eventually feel empowered. Because you can apply your new knowledge to your real situation and see results. It's kind of amazing.

One of the most important things you can do is open lines of communication and keep them open. Start therapy (both for your child and yourself) immediately. Don't wait. You can see different therapists, or the same one, together—it doesn't really matter. What *does* matter is that both you and your child are receiving professional guidance from an objective, qualified source.

If you can't afford to hire a therapist (you're definitely not alone here), there are alternatives. These include

- online chat forums,
- helpful apps,
- talking to your family doctor, and
- discussing your situation with other parents—you'll be surprised at how many of them are struggling as you are.

(Notice the common denominator is talking?) I include some resources for these alternatives after this chapter.

Here's the deal: when we go through a major upheaval with our kids, for some reason, we think we're alone. But we're not. There are enough people out there going through the same issues Cody and I were to warrant the sale of this book. It's like a miscarriage. Everyone thinks they're the only one, until you start to talk about it and find out most of the women you know have unfortunately gone through that very same experience.

In any case, the idea is to get both you and your teen (maybe the whole family, because a chronically anxious adolescent affects everyone around them—we're sensitive to the people we love) talking about what your teen—and you—are going through. As far as other ideas go, I have a few.

Here are my personal suggestions:

- Don't worry about actually understanding, because unless you've experienced anxiety yourself, you won't. Instead, be generally supportive. Be the person your child knows they can count on.
- Stay involved, keep communication lines open, and accept your child for who they are—because if no one does that, they will become lost. Teens who are going through chronic and crippling anxiety feel helpless, alone, afraid, and useless. Their self-esteem is negligible.
- Advocate for your child. Your kid will not do this for themselves—this one falls on the caregiver. *You.*

- Don't push or nag or threaten or go the tough love route—this will only make things worse. For someone with anxiety, being put on a schedule or timeline or being given ultimatums will probably only cause them to shut down even more. Instead, be patient, be supportive, and love them.
- Keep progress in perspective. It's very likely that you and your teen will experience the "two steps forward; one step back" thing. That's okay—it's still progress. Ultimately, you're looking for that upward swing. Sometimes it's helpful to look back three months and think about where they are now compared to where they were. Are they doing better or worse? Don't compare day to day; look back a month or two or three. Even a year.

## What Cody Wants Caregivers to Know

When I was the most anxious, I was really angry with my mom because she didn't understand what I was going through. My friends were there for me because I've always been there for them and because of the current culture of anxiety, everyone my age is familiar with it and understood what I was going through. They had patience for me—but my mom didn't (or it didn't seem like it, anyway).

What I want to say is this: don't give up on your kid. We don't know what we're doing, and we're scared and tired. I needed to feel secure, and I didn't because my mom kept making me leave our house. Although I understand now that she was scared too, and because of my behavior she felt like she had to make me leave, it still hurt, and I became even more scared and really mad.

We also didn't trust each other, and I felt like I had no one. The isolation is the worst—I just wanted everything to be normal and safe, and that needed to come from my mom because I didn't know how to make it better.

She was the grown-up, and I needed her to want to figure it out and help guide me.

## When Shit Goes Sideways

Sometimes, despite everything you do to help your teen, the problem becomes more than what you alone can handle. This is okay. This is normal, and this isn't your fault. It's *not* from lack of trying and doing your very best to help your teenager.

I promise.

Here are some possibilities to consider if or when the situation warrants it:

### Hospital Admission/External Intervention

This route would mainly be used for the following reasons:

- Extreme substance abuse
- Violence
- Self-harm (threatened or acted upon)
- Suicidality

Let's define these a little. Extreme substance abuse would essentially be an overdose or something close to that. It could also segue into the next reason for hospital admission, which is violence.

If your child is under the influence of drugs and alcohol and becomes violent, either to themselves or you or someone else, this is a good reason to call the police. It will not reflect badly on you to do so. You will not be—should not be—judged for wanting to protect yourself and your family. Also? It doesn't mean your teen is a bad person. It means they are hurting, have overmedicated, and need to be calmed by someone other than you.

It's that simple.

Knowing when you need immediate assistance from emergency responders, whether it be a policeman or paramedic, and making it happen, is one of the most difficult things parents can do. But it's also super important. Here's why:

- You can only do so much. You cannot do it all.
- Your child may need help that you are unable to provide. This is a difficult concept for parents. They may need the help of someone other than you.

- Your teen is a teen: sometimes they lie. If he's acting completely drunk and only claims to have had a drink or two, he's probably not telling the truth. (Were you completely honest with your parents about drinking when you were a teen?)

As parents, we feel the need to control what's going on with our children. We naturally and instinctively feel a great connection to both their successes and failures—but we need to remember that failures are learning experiences that cannot be learned if we're always sidestepping the result.

Here are some things to remember when navigating the tumultuous waters of teenage anxiety:

## Patience

I'll be the first to admit that I'm not a very patient person. I tend to view the world through the lens of logic and organizational planning—I *sucked* at initially supporting Cody with his anxiety.

But mood disorders are unpredictable and can be affected by so many things that are out of your (and your teen's) control. The secret is to let the concept of a "point A to point B" recovery go. It won't be easy. It won't be fast.

But it will happen, and patience actually makes it better.

## Love

I'd like to believe that a common thread throughout this book is love. Unconditional love is *everything* to a kid who's struggling with chronic anxiety that they don't understand. They are scared, they are young, and they need your love (and lots of it). Period. Relationship preservation is a must, so be sure to keep that in your foresight at all times. This doesn't mean catering to their anxious whims—this means giving them plenty of unconditional love while trying to communicate from a point of acceptance without judgment.

## Give Up Your Need to Control the Situation

I guess this goes with patience, but anxiety is not something you or anyone else (including your teen) can control. This is why you see mental health memes on Instagram that make fun of people who tell their friends with mood disorders to "hurry up and get better" or "just be normal." It's just not going to happen, for a huge variety of reasons. Give up the control you want to hold on to with this one. One, it won't work to think you may snag it, and two, it will make life easier for you if you understand that anxiety is definitely not something anyone can control.

It requires patience, love, and tools.

## Recovery and Coping Are Not Static and/or Predictable

Unfortunately, you won't be able to speed along your teen's recovery from anxiety and rush a desired outcome. I've learned this firsthand, and learning it was painful, so maybe just listen to what I'm telling you now and save yourself time and tons of frustration and heartache.

You kind of have to decide—make a decision now—not to set a timeline, a time frame, a calendar date, or anything else that you're tempted to label as a recovery date. I tried incentivizing, motivating, threatening, punishing, you name it. Nothing works, because your teen has no control over how they respond to an unfamiliar stimulus that decided to raid their body at random. So, no predictions. No goal dates.

This will only add extra pressure for both you and your teen, and I can guarantee that it probably won't work out the way you intend it.

## You Need Support

As in a network. You need a support network of family, friends, medical professionals (doctors, therapists, massage therapists, chiropractors), and probably the local gym to get you through this. Don't be afraid to talk about what you're going through—others are going through it, too.

If you've been hesitant to mention your teen's anxiousness to anyone for fear of being looked at sideways or your child being judged, or any other reason, you don't have to feel that way, and you should start talking.

This is hard. You need support, and so does your teenager.

## Create a Chart of Helpful Tips

Here is a quick summary of what is displayed on Anxiety Canada's website;[1] it contains some helpful tips that can guide you throughout this journey. Consider writing this down somewhere you can often reference, as I guarantee you'll need reminders.

- **Listen:** Make sure you take the time to listen to your teen's thoughts and feelings. Simply feeling heard can be very helpful for them.
- **Normalize:** It's important to let your teenager know that they are not alone. Lots of adolescents struggle with anxiety, with upward of 20 percent of them being diagnosed with an anxiety disorder during their lifetime.
- **Educate:** Let your teen know that anxiety is common and become experts on anxiety together.
- **Model:** Model facing fears by doing some of the feared challenges yourself, or even tackling your own fears. This can help to provide support and reassurance. Motivate your child through supportive coaching but be careful not to push your teen too far, too fast. Let them work at their own pace.
- **Tolerate:** Resist giving excessive reassurance, or letting your child avoid challenges or escape scary situations. While it's hard to see your child feeling anxious, learning to cope with anxiety is a critical life skill.[2]

## Cody and Teen Support

Schools should have safe spaces for suffering teens, including counseling services. Kids with anxiety aren't usually open to talking about anxiety because ironically, anxiety makes them think about being anxious. Teachers or important people in their lives should make discussion and self-care more mainstream.

Meditation, exercise, and focusing on one's own health without outside pressures is key to feeling better and thinking more clearly. Thinking about what you can do in the moment to make better choices should be emphasized, so mindfulness training would be helpful.

It's hard, but teenagers need to be trained to think more about the future as opposed to now when making choices and everyday decisions. These are topics of discussion that would be helpful to have around the dinner table.

## Love, Love, and More Love

When all is said and done, my thoughts land here: anxious teens who experience consistent support from their family and friends do better. Going to therapy (if you can get them there) works. Food and sleep make a massive impact on day-to-day function and mood. Communication is imperative. Acceptance and hard work go a long, long way.

And love, as always, is the answer.

Nobody has ever said, "I loved my kid too much." No kid has ever uttered, "All this love sucks." Love is hard, and even harder when combined with uncertainty, fear, and confusion. But it's still possible, still necessary, and still makes the biggest impact.

I came across an anonymous quote while writing this book that read, "And if those children are unresponsive, maybe you can't teach them yet, but you can love them. And if you love them today, maybe you can teach them tomorrow."

Ultimately, we need to find a way to identify our teens' emotional needs, address the issues we can spot quickly, and create a system of support for our kids so they don't become a statistic we could have prevented. If this is the age of anxiety and depression and stress and panic, then we must recognize it and figure out how to work with it in a way that is helpful for our teenagers and doesn't entice fear and fatigue.

It's up to us to pay attention and continue to guide our big kids because even though they may be tall and able and act relatively mature, we know they aren't ready to make adult decisions and react in a way that would indicate full brain formation. Our teens are still kids, and we're still their caregivers.

We need to give care.

In addition to you and your teen, the entire family needs extra special care, too. Anxiety affects everyone in the household, not only the anxious teen and their primary caregiver but everyone else who's around to feel the change in energy. Younger children may have less of their parents' attention due to the redirection of attention and concern. Your partner will feel the difference in energy application.

The whole family feels the shift—which can put even more pressure on *you* to allocate your resources in a different way. Bottom line? It's exhausting, and I know you're tired.

Hang in there.

## What You Can Do for You

Yes—I mean the caregiver. The mom, the dad, the aunt, the grandmother, the brother. The one who is shouldering the constant stress of trying to help their teenager who struggles with anxiety. (And probably depression.)

I'm talking about *you*.

You need care, too. If you're going to teach your teen how to care for themselves, you need to show by example. This means doing the very same things you want your teen to do: taking walks, getting in exercise, eating healthfully, meditating, trying to maintain a consistent sleep schedule. Conscious breathing, taking advantage of therapy, talking to good friends about what you're going through. Informing your family doctor. Educating yourself on the topic of anxiety and depression. Keeping open lines of communication between yourself and your teen.

Showing yourself love and respect, because kids learn through example.

It means knowing when you need a break and taking that break. As a parent or caregiver, we tend to put our family's needs ahead of our own. (Mothers especially seem to be hardwired for this.) But when someone suffering from chronic anxiety resides in your home and is under your care, we need to retrain ourselves to know when it's time to take a step back.

You cannot help another thrive if you yourself are not thriving.

My last words for you to consider, which were given to me by a close friend at a time when I needed them most, are these: you are doing the best you know how, right now. We're humans, and we grow and learn and expand our brains in astonishing ways and rates. You may know better now than you did last month.

But last month, you were doing the best you knew how at *that* time.

And now, maybe you're doing even better. Don't regret how you handled something with your teen last month or last year. As parents and caregivers with high emotional investments in our children's health and well-being, you need to know that whatever happened or is happening right now, you did your best, and you are *still* doing your best.

You're not alone, just as your teen is not alone. You are loved, just as your teen is loved.

Everything will be okay.

## Chapter Summary

Until this point, this book has been about how you can help your teen battle their chronic anxiety. But this last chapter was for you, the caregiver. Here is a summary of points for you to refer to that can help you help yourself:

- Find people to talk to about what you're going through.
- Check out the resources at the end of this book, and seek professional support if you feel it's necessary.
- Remember to listen, normalize, educate, model, and tolerate.
- Know you're doing the best you can.
- Love yourself as you love your teen.
- Remember to take care of *you*.

# RESOURCES

THERE are various types of resources that both caregivers and teens may be interested in checking out. For many of us, the obvious choice for support is to seek out a qualified therapist or mental health professional, but in reality, most of us can't afford to pay privately for one-on-one sessions.

Luckily, there are several inexpensive and free resources we can pull from to obtain help in dealing with teenage anxiety. These include . . .

## Smartphone Apps

Mental health apps offer a wealth of resources that make therapeutic techniques more accessible, portable, and cost-effective. Within minutes, you can find and download innumerable apps that incorporate proven techniques such as cognitive behavioral therapy (CBT) and acceptance commitment therapy (ACT). They can address everything from depression to eating disorder recovery, anxiety, bipolar disorder, obsessive-compulsive disorder, and more.

I personally hadn't even considered apps to be something that had the potential to be helpful until the idea was recommended in a workshop that I took in the fall of 2018 at the Surrey International Writers Conference. The workshop was called *Writing with Mental Health Issues*, created by published author Alyssa Cole.

While the majority of these apps are admittedly lacking peer-reviewed research to support their claims, health experts predict that they will play an important role in the future of mental health care by providing innovative solutions for the self-management of mental health disorders.

Here are a few apps for your teen to try; all are free and available on iOS and Android:

- **MindShift:** One of the best mental health apps designed specifically for teens and young adults with anxiety. Rather than trying to avoid anxious feelings, MindShift stresses the importance of changing how your teen thinks about anxiety.
- **Self-Help for Anxiety Management (SAM):** Might be perfect for your teenager if they're interested in self-help but meditation isn't entirely their thing. Users of the app are prompted to build their own twenty-four-hour anxiety toolkit that allows them to track anxious thoughts and behavior over time and learn twenty-five different self-help techniques. Your teen can also use SAM's "Social Cloud" feature to confidentially connect with other users in a supportive online community for additional support.
- **CBT Thought Record Diary:** Your teen can use CBT Thought Record Diary to document negative emotions, analyze flaws in their thinking, and reevaluate their thoughts. This is a great app for gradually changing your teen's approach to anxiety-inducing situations and their thinking patterns for future situations.
- **Calm:** This app provides people experiencing stress and anxiety with guided meditations, sleep stories, breathing programs, and relaxing music. This app is truly universal and is helpful whether your teen has never tried meditation before or practices regularly.

## Phone Numbers

- **Emergency Services:** Dial 911 for teens who are threatening self-harm.
- **Crisis Text Line:** Text CONNECT to 741741 in the United States.

## Online Support

- **Crisis Text Hotline:** crisistextline.org/anxiety
- **Teen Anxiety Support Group:** dailystrength.org/group/teen-anxiety
- **TeenHelp.com:** teenhelp.com/stress-anxiety/teen-anxiety
- **The Tribe Wellness Community:** support.therapytribe.com/teen-support-group

## Reading Material

The following selection of reading material helped me immensely when attempting to navigate the world of anxiety with Cody:

### Books:

- *The Beating Anxiety Workbook* by Dr. Stephanie Fitzgerald
- *Guilt, Shame, and Anxiety* by Peter R. Breggin, MD
- *Discipline without Damage* by Dr. Vanessa Lapointe
- *Anxiety* by Joseph LeDoux
- *The 10 Best Anxiety Busters* by Dr. Margaret Wehrenberg

### Online:

- **Anxiety Canada:** anxietycanada.com
- **Anxiety and Depression Association of America:** adaa.org

## Miscellaneous

- **Find a Therapist Directory (Anxiety and Depression Association of America):** members.adaa.org/page/FATMain
- **Being You Parent Viewing Guide:** understood.org/-/media/b106360d9b21441db9de330ac713c995.pdf

# ABOUT THE AUTHORS

**Jennifer Browne** is the author of six wellness books, including *Happy Healthy Gut*, *Vegetarian Comfort Foods*, *The Good Living Guide to Medicinal Tea*, *Baby Nosh*, and *The Anti-Anxiety Cookbook*. She lives with her three kids and golden retriever in Abbotsford, British Columbia. Visit her website at jenniferbrowne.ca.

**Cody Buchanan** is the coauthor of this book and has had long-term personal experience with chronic anxiety. As a young teen, he suffered in silence for years, and he was sixteen before his condition became apparent to others, almost nineteen before treatment commenced. Buchanan is the oldest son of Jennifer Browne and agreed to participate in this project to help others better understand their anxious family members.

# ACKNOWLEDGMENTS

CODY and I would like to thank everyone who helped this book become a reality. It began as an idea to help us communicate more effectively about Cody's chronic and often debilitating anxiety. I thought I could use the research I'd been already immersed in, and he would gain a voice to discuss his experiences. This all happened and more—writing this was an amazing opportunity for the both of us.

Many thanks to Dr. Vanessa Lapointe for agreeing to provide a foreword that would give me goosebumps when I read it and to Judy Arnold and Maya Coleman for providing constructive feedback before we submitted the project.

Thank you especially to Dr. Carla Dassinger, who served as a professional consultant to us throughout the writing process. We couldn't be more grateful for her patience, knowledge, genuine interest, and generosity.

Thanks also to both Abigail and Nicole, Skyhorse editors, who loved the idea behind the book enough to get excited about it.

# INDEX

# ENDNOTES

1. Anxiety and Depression Association of America, https://adaa.org/about-adaa/press-room/facts-statistics#.

## Chapter 1: An Anxious Generation

1. Benoit Denizet-Lewis, "Why Are More American Teenagers than Ever Suffering from Severe Anxiety?," *New York Times Magazine*, October 11, 2017, https://www.nytimes.com/2017/10/11/magazine/why-are-more-american-teenagers-than-ever-suffering-from-severe-anxiety.html.
2. Katherine Martinelli et al., *Understanding Anxiety in Children and Teens: 2018 Children's Mental Health Report* (Child Mind Institute, 2018), https://www.cmhnetwork.org/wp-content/uploads/2018/10/CMI_2018CMHR.pdf.
3. Peter Breggin, *Guilt, Shame, and Anxiety: Understanding and Overcoming Negative Emotions.* (Prometheus Books, 2014), 175. Amherst, New York.
4. Ibid.
5. Denizet-Lewis, "Why Are More."
6. M. Anderson and J. Jiang, *Teens, Social Media, and Technology 2018*, May 31, 2018, http://www.pewinternet.org/wp-content/uploads/sites/9/2018/05/PI_2018.05.31_TeensTech_FINAL.pdf.
7. Ibid.
8. Heather Cleland Woods and Holly Scott, "#Sleepyteens: Social Media Use in Adolescence Is Associated with Poor Sleep Quality, Anxiety, Depression and Low Self-Esteem," *Journal of Adolescence*, no. 51 (August 1, 2016): 41–49, https://doi.org/10.1016/j.adolescence.2016.05.008.
9. Rachel Ehmke, "How Using Social Media Affects Teenagers," Child Mind Institute, https://childmind.org/article/how-using-social-media-affects-teenagers/.

10. Kevin McSpadden, "You Now Have a Shorter Attention Span Than a Goldfish," *Time*, May 14, 2015, http://time.com/3858309/attention-spans-goldfish/.
11. Ibid.
12. Martinelli et al., *Understanding Anxiety*.
13. Catherine Steiner-Adair and Teresa H. Barker, *The Big Disconnect* (Harper, 2013). New York, NY.
14. Ehmke, "How Using Social Media."
15. National Institute of Mental Health, "Any Anxiety Disorder," last updated November 2017, https://www.nimh.nih.gov/health/statistics/any-anxiety-disorder.shtml.
16. Ibid.
17. Ibid.
18. Ibid.
19. Martinelli et al., *Understanding Anxiety*.
20. Ibid.
21. Ibid.
22. Ibid.

## Chapter 2: Symptoms and Types of Anxiety

1. Denizet-Lewis, "Why Are More."
2. Breggin, *Guilt, Shame, and Anxiety*, 145.
3. Emily Waters, "10 Quick and Effective Ways to Nip Your Anxiety in the Bud," PsychCentral, last updated October 8, 2018, https://psychcentral.com/lib/10-quick-and-effective-ways-to-nip-your-anxiety-in-the-bud/.
4. "Grounding Exercises," Living Well, https://www.livingwell.org.au/well-being/mental-health/grounding-exercises.
5. Anxiety and Depression Association of America, "Generalized Anxiety Disorder (GAD), 2019. Web. https://adaa.org/understanding-anxiety/generalized-anxiety-disorder-gad.
6. Elizabeth I. Martin et al., "The Neurobiology of Anxiety Disorders: Brain Imaging, Genetics, and Psychoneuroendocrinology," *Psychiatric Clinics of North America* 32, no. 3 (September 2009): 549–75, https://doi.org/10.1016/j.psc.2009.05.004.
7. "Facts and Statistics," Anxiety and Depression Association of America, https://adaa.org/about-adaa/press-room/facts-statistics#.
8. Martinelli et al., *Understanding Anxiety*.
9. Ibid.
10. Murray et al., *Anxiety and Stress Disorders*, 21.
11. "Facts and Statistics."

12. Kristy L. Dalrymple and Mark Zimmerman, "Age of Onset of Social Anxiety Disorder in Depressed Outpatients," *Journal of Anxiety Disorders* 25, no. 1 (January 1, 2011): 131–37, https://doi.org/10.1016/j.janxdis.2010.08.012.
13. "Facts and Statistics."
14. National Center for Biotechnology Information, "Nine Substance-Induced Disorders," http://www.ncbi.nlm.nih.gov/books/NBK64178/.

## Chapter 3: The Teenage Brain

1. Sarah-Jayne Blakemore, Stephanie Burnett, and Ronald E Dahl, "The Role of Puberty in the Developing Adolescent Brain," *Human Brain Mapping* 31, no. 6 (June 2010): 926–33, https://doi.org/10.1002/hbm.21052.
2. Vanessa Lapointe, *Discipline without Damage* (Life Tree Media, 2016), 19. Vancouver, BC.
3. Russell D. Romeo, "The Teenage Brain: The Stress Response and the Adolescent Brain," *Current Directions in Psychological Science* 22, no. 2 (April 2013): 140–45, https://doi.org/10.1177/0963721413475445.
4. Douglas S. Mennin et al., "Is Generalized Anxiety Disorder an Anxiety or Mood Disorder? Considering Multiple Factors as We Ponder the Fate of GAD," *Depression and Anxiety* 25, no. 4 (2008): 289–99, https://doi.org/10.1002/da.20493.
5. Katja Beesdo et al., "Incidence of Social Anxiety Disorder and the Consistent Risk for Secondary Depression in the First Three Decades of Life," *Archives of General Psychiatry* 64, no. 8 (August 1, 2007): 903–12, https://doi.org/10.1001/archpsyc.64.8.903.
6. Martinelli et al., *Understanding Anxiety.*
7. Kristy L. Dalrymple and Mark Zimmerman, "Age of Onset of Social Anxiety Disorder in Depressed Outpatients," *Journal of Anxiety Disorders* 25, no. 1 (January 1, 2011): 131–37, https://doi.org/10.1016/j.janxdis.2010.08.012.
8. Lapointe, *Discipline without Damage*, 40.

## Chapter 4: Genetics, Stress, and Anxiety

1. Martinelli et al., *Understanding Anxiety.*
2. Denise Griswold, "Introduction to Inherited Anxiety," Calm Clinic, October 28, 2018, https://www.calmclinic.com/anxiety/causes/inheriting.
3. Ibid.
4. Lisa Y. Maeng and Mohammed R. Milad, "Sex Differences in Anxiety Disorders: Interactions between Fear, Stress, and Gonadal Hormones," 2015. Web. https://www.ncbi.nlm.nih.gov/pmc/articles/PMC4823998/.
5. M.A. Waszczuk, H.M.S. Zavos, and T.C. Eley. "Genetic and Environmental Influences on Relationship Between Anxiety Sensitivity and Anxiety Subscales

in Children," Pubmed, 2013. Web. https://www.ncbi.nlm.nih.gov/pmc/articles/PMC3878378/.
6. Meghan Crosby Budinger, Tess K. Drazdowski, and Golda S. Ginsburg, "Anxiety-Promoting Parenting Behaviors: A Comparison of Anxious Parents with and without Social Anxiety Disorder," *Child Psychiatry & Human Development* 44, no. 3 (June 2013): 412–18, https://doi.org/10.1007/s10578-012-0335-9.
7. "Social Anxiety Disorder: Recognition, Assessment and Treatment," https://www.ncbi.nlm.nih.gov/books/NBK327674/. NICE Clinical Guidelines, No. 159. National Collaborating Centre for Mental Health (UK). Leicester (UK): British Psychological Society; 2013.
8. Boadie W. Dunlop and Charles B. Nemeroff, "The Role of Dopamine in the Pathophysiology of Depression," *Archives of General Psychiatry* 64, no. 3 (March 2007): 327–37, https://doi.org/10.1001/archpsyc.64.3.327.
9. American Psychological Association, *Stress in America: Are Teens Adopting Adults' Stress Habits?* (American Psychological Association, 2014), https://www.apa.org/news/press/releases/stress/2013/stress-report.pdf.
10. Ibid.
11. Fiza Pirani, "Why More US Teens Are Suffering From Severe Anxiety Than Ever Before—and How Parents Can Help," *Atlanta Journal Constitution*, updated October 10, 2018, https://www.ajc.com/news/health-med-fit-science/why-more-teens-are-suffering-from-severe-anxiety-than-ever-before-and-how-parents-can-help/cFlF86X6Qvn9IHqBX75jzK/.

## Chapter 5: Head Injuries and Mental Health

1. Jonathan M. Silver et al., "The Association between Head Injuries and Psychiatric Disorders: Findings from the New Haven NIMH Epidemiologic Catchment Area Study," *Brain Injury* 15, no. 11 (January 1, 2001): 935–45, https://doi.org/10.1080/02699050110065295.
2. "Concussions," Cleveland Clinic, last reviewed January 2, 2015, https://my.clevelandclinic.org/health/diseases/15038-concussions.
3. "Brain Injury Patterns Linked to Post-Concussion Depression and Anxiety," Radiological Society of North America, June 16, 2015, https://press.rsna.org/timssnet/media/pressreleases/14_pr_target.cfm?ID=815.
4. American Academy of Neurology, "After a Concussion, Which Teens Will Have Emotional Symptoms?," ScienceDaily, July 10, 2014, https://www.sciencedaily.com/releases/2014/07/140710161523.htm.
5. "CDC Initiative: Concussion in Sports and Play," Practical Pain Management, last updated May 8, 2014, https://www.practicalpainmanagement.com/pain/headache/post-trauma-headache/cdc-initiative-concussion-sports-play.

6. Daniel H. Daneshvar et al., "Long Term Consequences: Effects on Normal Development Profile after Concussion," *Physical Medicine and Rehabilitation Clinics of North America* 22, no. 4 (November 2011): 683–700, https://doi.org/10.1016/j.pmr.2011.08.009.

## Chapter 6: Anxiety and Education

1. John Kelly, "Anxiety in Schools," *Brainstorm Blog* (blog), Child Mind Institute, September 26, 2018, https://childmind.org/blog/anxiety-in-schools-nasp-2018-childrens-mental-health-report/.
2. "Types of Anxiety in Children," Child Mind Institute, https://childmind.org/guide/a-teachers-guide-to-anxiety-in-the-classroom/kinds-of-anxiety/.
3. Kelly, "Anxiety in Schools."
4. Habil Gil Noam, "How Do We Help Students Feel Safe in School Again?," *Psychology Today*, May 24, 2018, https://www.psychologytoday.com/us/blog/the-inner-life-students/201805/how-do-we-help-students-feel-safe-in-school-again.

## Chapter 8: Anxiety and Gut Health

1. "Facts about IBS," International Foundation for Gastrointestinal Disorders, last updated November 24, 2016, https://www.aboutibs.org/facts-about-ibs.html.

## Chapter 9: Natural Ways to Help Your Teen Cope

1. Quincy Seale, "Seven Natural Supplements for Anxiety That Work," KeepInspiringMe.com, https://www.keepinspiring.me/7-natural-supplements-for-anxiety-that-work/.
2. Antonia N. Kaczkurkin and Edna B. Foa, "Cognitive-Behavioral Therapy for Anxiety Disorders: An Update on the Empirical Evidence," *Dialogues in Clinical Neuroscience* 17, no. 3 (September 2015): 337–46.
3. Poppy L. A. Schoenberg and Anthony S. David, "Biofeedback for Psychiatric Disorders: A Systematic Review," *Applied Psychophysiology and Biofeedback* 39, no. 2 (June 2014): 109–35, https://doi.org/10.1007/s10484-014-9246-9.
4. Robert Reiner, "Integrating a Portable Biofeedback Device into Clinical Practice for Patients with Anxiety Disorders: Results of a Pilot Study," *Applied Psychophysiology and Biofeedback* 33, no. 1 (March 2008): 55–61, https://doi.org/10.1007/s10484-007-9046-6.
5. "Yoga for Anxiety and Depression," *Harvard Mental Health Letter*, last updated May 9, 2018, https://www.health.harvard.edu/mind-and-mood/yoga-for-anxiety-and-depression.

6. "Ten Things Parents Can Do to Prevent Suicide," HealthyChildren.org, last updated January 17, 2019, https://www.healthychildren.org/English/health-issues/conditions/emotional-problems/Pages/Ten-Things-Parents-Can-Do-to-Prevent-Suicide.aspx.
7. "Yoga for Anxiety and Depression."
8. Alice Walton, "Mind-Body Practices Like Meditation and Yoga Help Teens with Anxiety, Study Finds," *Forbes*, July 28, 2018, https://www.forbes.com/sites/alicegwalton/2018/07/28/mind-body-practices-like-meditation-and-yoga-help-teens-with-anxiety-study-finds/#5ef8d72a11df.
9. Jhaneel Lockhart and Melanie Hicken, "Fourteen Executives Who Swear by Meditation," *Business Insider*, May 9, 2012, https://www.businessinsider.com/ceos-who-meditate-2012-5?op=1.
10. Dorene Petersen, "Anxious or Feeling Down? Can Essential Oils Help?," *ACHS Holistic Health and Wellness Blog* (blog), January 27, 2017, http://info.achs.edu/blog/depression-and-anxiety-can-essential-oils-help.
11. H. Woelk and S. Schläfke, "A Multi-Center, Double-Blind, Randomised Study of the Lavender Oil Preparation Silexan in Comparison to Lorazepam for Generalized Anxiety Disorder," *Phytomedicine: International Journal of Phytotherapy and Phytopharmacology* 17, no. 2 (February 2010): 94–99, https://doi.org/10.1016/j.phymed.2009.10.006.
12. Farzaneh Barati et al., "The Effect of Aromatherapy on Anxiety in Patients," *Nephro-Urology Monthly* 8, no. 5 (July 31, 2016), https://doi.org/10.5812/numonthly.38347.
13. Shaheen E. Lakhan and Karen F. Vieira, "Nutritional and Herbal Supplements for Anxiety and Anxiety-Related Disorders: Systematic Review," *Nutrition Journal* 9 (October 7, 2010): 42, https://doi.org/10.1186/1475-2891-9-42.
14. Lakhan and Vieira, "Nutritional and Herbal Supplements."
15. Robert J. Hedaya, "Vitamin B12," *Psychology Today*, February 2, 2012, https://www.psychologytoday.com/us/blog/health-matters/201202/vitamin-b12.
16. Ivaldo Jesus Lima de Oliveira et al., "Effects of Oral Vitamin C Supplementation on Anxiety in Students: A Double-Blind, Randomized, Placebo-Controlled Trial," *Pakistan Journal of Biological Sciences* 18, no. 1 (January 2015): 11–18.
17. Stacy Horn, "Singing Changes Your Brain," *Time*, August 16, 2013, http://ideas.time.com/2013/08/16/singing-changes-your-brain/.
18. Ibid.
19. James Lake, "Kava Is an Effective and Safe Treatment of Anxiety," *Psychology Today*, March 15, 2017, https://www.psychologytoday.com/ca/blog/integrative-mental-health-care/201703/kava-is-effective-and-safe-treatment-anxiety.

20. Peter Bongiorno, "Ashwaganda for Anxiety," *Psychology Today*, January 8, 2014, https://www.psychologytoday.com/ca/blog/inner-source/201401/ashwaganda-anxiety.
21. "Rhodiola Rosea," Mental Health America, http://www.mentalhealthamerica.net/rhodiola-rosea.
22. Lakhan and Vieira, "Nutritional and Herbal Supplements."
23. "An Emotional Support Animal Can Help with Anxiety," Anxiety.org, March 18, 2014, https://www.anxiety.org/emotional-support-animals-help-anxiety.
24. Helen Brooks et al., "Ontological Security and Connectivity Provided by Pets: A Study in the Self-Management of the Everyday Lives of People Diagnosed with a Long-Term Mental Health Condition," *BMC Psychiatry* 16, no. 1 (December 9, 2016): 409, https://doi.org/10.1186/s12888-016-1111-3.

## Chapter 10: Medication for Anxiety

1. Raychelle Cassada Lohmann, "Understanding Teen Anxiety," *Psychology Today*, February 14, 2015, https://www.psychologytoday.com/ca/blog/teen-angst/201502/understanding-teen-anxiety.
2. Tarang Sharma et al., "Suicidality and Aggression during Antidepressant Treatment: Systematic Review and Meta-Analyses Based on Clinical Study Reports," *BMJ*, 352 (January 27, 2016): i65, https://doi.org/10.1136/bmj.i65.
3. Mayo Clinic staff, "Selective Serotonin Reuptake Inhibitors (SSRIs)," Mayo Clinic, May 17, 2018, https://www.mayoclinic.org/diseases-conditions/depression/in-depth/ssris/art-20044825.
4. Mayo Clinic staff, "Serotonin and Norepinephrine Reuptake Inhibitors (SNRIs)," Mayo Clinic, June 21, 2016, https://www.mayoclinic.org/diseases-conditions/depression/in-depth/antidepressants/art-20044970.
5. Craig Freudenrich, "How Antidepressants Work," HowStuffWorks.com, September 20, 2007, https://science.howstuffworks.com/life/antidepressant4.htm.
6. "Big Pharma: Are They Advertising Addiction?," DrugAbuse.com, https://drugabuse.com/big-pharma-are-they-advertising-addiction/.
7. Kathleen Smith, "Anxiety Medications for Teens: Treatment Options for Your Child," Psycom.net, last updated May 29, 2018, https://www.psycom.net/anxiety-medications-teenagers.

## Chapter 11: Self-Harm and Suicide

1. Harold S. Koplewicz, "Antidepressants and Teen Suicides," Child Mind Institute, https://childmind.org/article/antidepressants-and-teen-suicides/.
2. Janis Whitlock, John Eckenrode, and Daniel Silverman, "Self-Injurious Behaviors in a College Population," *Pediatrics* 117, no. 6 (June 2006): 1939–48, https://doi.org/10.1542/peds.2005–2543.

3. Samantha Gluck, "Self Injury, Self Harm Statistics and Facts," HealthyPlace.com, last updated August 26, 2016, https://www.healthyplace.com/abuse/self-injury/self-injury-self-harm-statistics-and-facts.
4. Ibid.
5. "Ten Things Parents Can Do."
6. Josh Nepon et al., "The Relationship Between Anxiety Disorders and Suicide Attempts: Findings from the National Epidemiologic Survey on Alcohol and Related Conditions," *Depression and Anxiety* 27, no. 9 (September 2010): 791–98, https://doi.org/10.1002/da.20674.
7. Ibid.
8. National Institute of Mental Health, *Suicide in America: Frequently Asked Questions* (Bethesda, MD: National Institute of Mental Health, 2018), https://www.nimh.nih.gov/health/publications/suicide-faq/suicideinamericafaq-508_149986.pdf.
9. James Bolton et al., "Use of Alcohol and Drugs to Self-Medicate Anxiety Disorders in a Nationally Representative Sample," *Journal of Nervous and Mental Disease* 194, no. 11 (November 2006): 818–25, https://doi.org/10.1097/01.nmd.0000244481.63148.98.
10. Mayo Clinic staff, "Selective Serotonin Reuptake Inhibitors."
11. "Ten Things Parents Can Do."
12. Mayo Clinic staff, "Selective Serotonin Reuptake Inhibitors."
13. Ibid.
14. "Ten Things Parents Can Do."
15. Mayo Clinic staff, "Selective Serotonin Reuptake Inhibitors."

## Chapter 12: Care for the Caregiver

1. Anxiety Canada, https://www.anxietycanada.com.
2. Ibid.

# NOTES

# NOTES

# NOTES

# NOTES

# NOTES

# NOTES